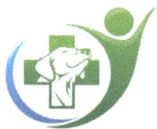

![First Aid for Pets.net logo]

First Aid for **Pets**.net

The contents of this book could save your pet's life!

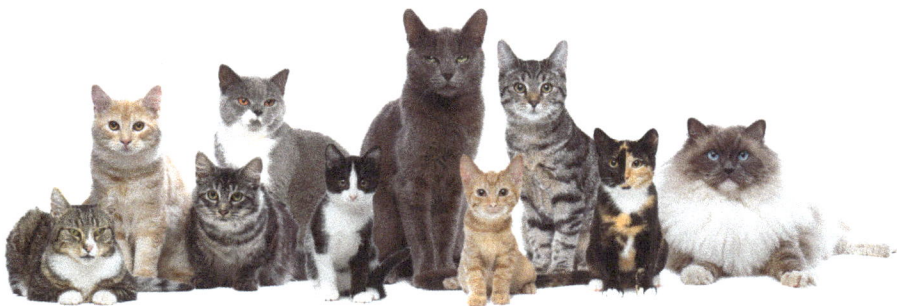

Introduction

This guide is designed for all cat lovers. It will explain how to help your pet or any other cat should an accident happen. It is ideal for those working with cats and pet owners to gain the skills and confidence to help in an emergency until veterinary support is available.

The manual takes you through a step-by-step guide to examining your pet, recognising if there is something wrong and treatment for common veterinary emergencies.

The book covers most common first aid emergencies, including helping a choking cat, cat bites, car accidents, injured limbs, CPR, fitting and poisoning.

The content conforms to the RECOVER guidelines for veterinary CPR and complies with the Veterinary Care Act.

The manual is designed to give you the knowledge to help your pet should an accident happen and is ideal for those working with cats and pet owners to gain the skills and confidence to help in an emergency until veterinary support is available. You will learn vital skills such as recognising when there is something seriously wrong. Learning how to take a cat's pulse and do CPR if necessary. Recognition and treatment for other common

First Aid emergencies, including bites, how to help your choking cat, assist if they are hit by a car, bandage bleeding and injured limbs, seizures, poisoning and much more.

The manual consists of illustrated step by step directions, flow charts, diagrams and accompanies the comprehensive online First Aid for Cats course available from:
http://www.firstaidforpets.net

It is impossible to cover all eventualities within this course, or to equip you with the knowledge and skills to appropriately diagnose and treat in unpredictable real-life situations. If you suspect illness or injury, you should always seek immediate professional medical advice.

The Author has made every effort to ensure the accuracy of the information contained within the course, however this course is merely a guide and the Author does not accept any liability or responsibility for any inaccuracies or for any mistreatment or misdiagnosis of any person or animal, however caused.

The course material has been written by Emma Hammett, Qualified Nurse, First Aid Trainer and founder of First Aid for Life in conjunction with other medical, first aid, animal and veterinary professionals. If you have any queries concerning this course, please contact:
emma@firstaidforlife.org.uk

Contents

Introduction..........................2

Role of the first aider

Safety and Consent 4
Priorities of Treatment..............6
Know your cat - 7
Top to Tail Survey......................7
What the Vet needs to know 10
First Aid Kits..............................12
How to muzzle a cat...............15

Emergency life-saving actions

Primary Survey 18
Recovery Position.....................23
Resuscitation: CPR (Cardio Pulmonary Resuscitation) 24
Choking..26
Drowning 30

Wounds and bleeding

Wounds and Bleeding 31
Types of bleeding 32
Treatment of bleeding............33
Embedded objects...................36
Splinters 37
Nosebleeds................................38
Bite wounds...............................39
Eye Injuries................................40

Shock 41
Road traffic accidents - how to help 44

Medical emergencies

Allergic reaction 47
Bites and Stings........................50
Burns...54
Electric shock 58
Poisoning 61
Common poisons – human food..64
Common poisons - non -foods 68
Breaks and Dislocations.........70
Head Injuries..............................73
Spinal Injuries 74
Seizures.......................................75

Extremes of body temperature

Extremes of body temperature 78
Heat Stroke 81
Hypothermia..............................82

Useful advice

When is it an emergency?.....84
Caring for a neonate...............86
Behavioural changes..............94

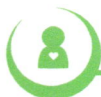

Safety and Consent

You should always start by checking for DANGER – you don't know what has injured them and if you are injured as well, you won't be able to help them.

Human safety ALWAYS takes priority over that of the animal. If at any point you are concerned for your own safety, you should not approach the animal, and just get help.

The priority with any first aid situation is to ensure your own safety and that of the injured animal. If an animal is hurt, you would ideally keep them still and avoid moving them. However, if an animal has been injured on the road, it may be necessary to remove them to somewhere safe where they can be treated. Ideally this would be done very carefully and often a car parcel shelf can prove extremely useful as a makeshift stretcher. If a cat travel carrier is available, even better.

Always approach an injured cat with extreme caution, even if it is your pet and you know them well. When an animal is in pain, they tend to behave differently and could bite or hurt you. Avoid looking an animal straight in the eyes as they can find this intimidating.

Be as calm as possible and avoid shouting or making sudden movements. Keep the injured animal warm and dry and move them as little as possible.
When an animal is injured it is often instinctive for them to find somewhere to hide. Do your best to be as calm and reassuring as possible so that they do not feel the urge to try and move themselves and escape.

Consider muzzling the animal if there is a strong risk of them biting, even the most placid of animals will bite if they are scared or hurt. However, never muzzle them if they are having any difficulty breathing.

It can be difficult muzzling a cat as they have such short noses. However, using something like

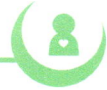

a pillowcase to cover them, can calm them and make it easier for you to transport or treat them with less risk of them scratching or biting you.

You need to keep yourself safe the whole time, ensure that in addition to a check at the beginning, keep checking and make sure you don't put yourself at risk at any point at all.

If you are thinking of resuscitating someone else's cat you should always ensure you have permission to do so. Giving CPR is likely to damage the cat's ribs and if they do survive, this could result in hefty Vet's bills.

TRY TO KEEP YOURSELF AND THE ANIMAL AS CALM AS POSSIBLE

ALWAYS KEEP THINGS AS SIMPLE AS YOU CAN - TREAT WHAT YOU SEE!

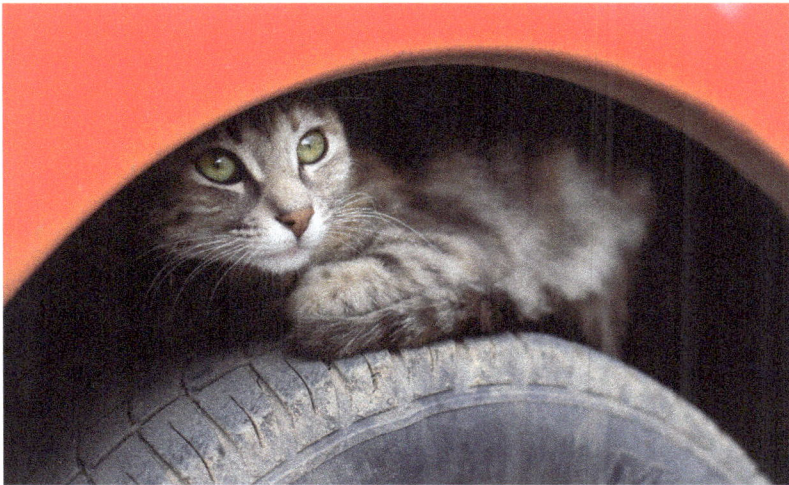

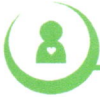

Priorities of Treatment

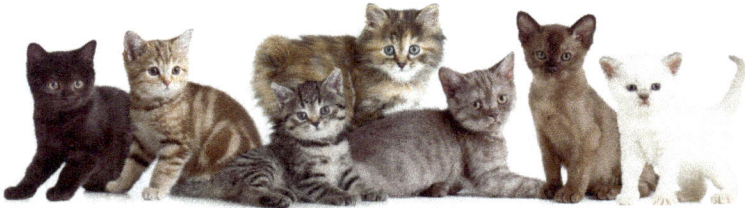

The key objectives when giving First Aid are to:

- Preserve Life

- Prevent the condition worsening

- Promote Recovery

When you are dealing with a serious incident whether with an animal or human; it is crucially important that you prioritize any life-threatening conditions and treat those first.

Breathing - This is your number one priority, if they are not breathing and you don't do anything about it they are dead!

Bleeding and Burns - Both life-threatening conditions. Providing the casualty is breathing, your next priority is to stop bleeding and treat burns – before being distracted by anything else.

Broken Bones - Are rarely life threatening - but can prove a distraction from more serious priorities.

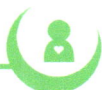

Know your cat - Top to Tail Survey

It is very helpful to think in advance about how you would manage a medical emergency and to have some baseline measurements so you can quickly recognise when there is something wrong.

Regularly practice conducting a top to toe examination on your pet. Start with the head and systematically work down. Build up to more sensitive areas such as their eyes and other areas they may not like being scrutinised. This is really important to help avoid your pet becoming alarmed if you need to properly examine them in an emergency situation. Regular examinations should make it easier for you to swiftly spot any abnormalities.

Normal range for the vital signs:

Temperature – 100.5 to 102.5 F or 38-39.3 C

Respiratory rate 10 – 30 per minute

Pulse rate 60-140bpm (smaller cats tend to have a faster pulse rate possibly up to 160 bpm, large cats tend to have a slower pulse rate 60-80bpm)

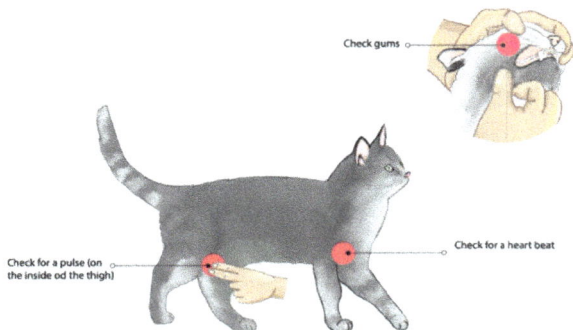

Check gums

Check for a pulse (on the inside od the thigh)

Check for a heart beat

feel the artery pulsing here (your thumb has a strong pulse itself so don't use this to take their pulse as otherwise you will be timing your own pulse rate).

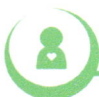

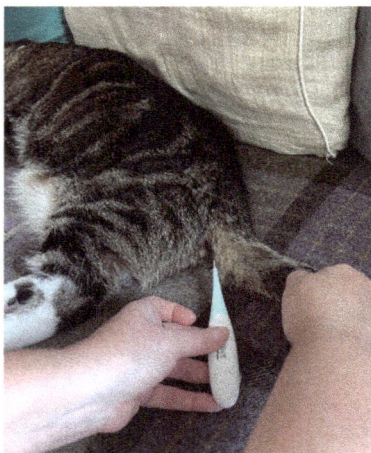

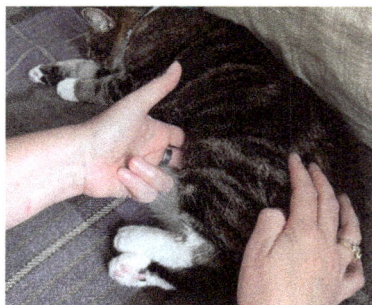

Taking your pet's temperature - The temperature can be taken using an ordinary digital or rectal thermometer lubricated with some olive oil and gently inserted into their anus with the end touching the inner wall of their anus. This is often easier to do when the animal is sitting, but if they are standing use your free hand to support their stomach and prevent them from sitting.

To take their pulse - The easiest place to find the cat's pulse is in the upper third of their thigh. Place your hand over the top of their thigh and gently squeeze your fingers just underneath their leg, you should be able to

The femoral pulse can be difficult to find on pets with a greater fat covering. You can also listen for a heartbeat. Time the pulse for 15 seconds and multiply the result by 4 to get the beats per minute.

To take their respiratory rate - Carefully watch the rise and fall of their chest and count the breaths for a 15 second period – multiply by 4 for the rate for 1 minute.

Checking mucosal membranes – their gums should be pinkish-red, smooth and moist – if they are not, they could be going into shock or showing signs of

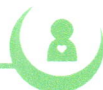

dehydration. Deep red sticky gums could be a sign of heat exhaustion.

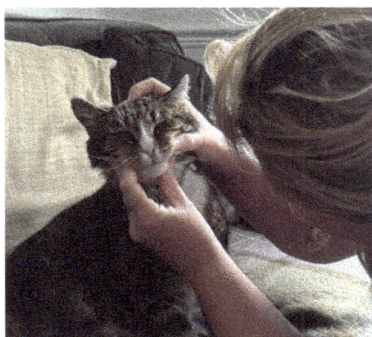

Capillary refill time – in a healthy animal if you push down on their gums quickly and then release your finger, the colour should return almost immediately in 1-2 seconds. The time it takes for the colour to return is known as the capillary refill time and a slowness for the colour to return could indicate that the animal is going into shock.

Helpful information for Pet owners to keep to hand:

• Veterinary Surgery number

• Name of Vet

• Cat's name and Breed

• Date of birth

• Gender

• Female cat - neutered?

• Weight

• Micro-chipping details

• Vaccination information

• Insurance details

• Medical conditions

• Medication

• Previous medical history

• Name of a local adult or neighbour known and trusted – to look after other pets in an emergency or to quickly come over and help

• Emergency Medication for your pet should be clearly marked and remain safe but accessible for urgent use.

If the animal is injured outside, it is important to try and insulated them from ground if at all possible and cover them to keep them warm. This is of particular importance in cold weather and it may be necessary to carefully move them to ensure they are warm and safe.

Ensure you have an appropriately stocked First Aid kit to hand.

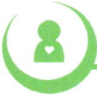

What the Vet needs to know

Always phone the Vet in advance so they can give you advice on stabilising and transporting your pet and to ensure they are open, available and the closest service to visit.

Your own Vet may not be closest in an emergency. Apps are available to download onto your phone to help you to locate your nearest Vet.

Make sure you have a fully charged mobile phone with you, keep your Vet's phone number to hand and name of the practice.

It is advisable to phone the Practice before you leave as they are likely to be able to suggest additional First Aid that you can do in order to stabilise the animal before bringing them in.

Ideally keep the injured animal as calm and still as you can, only move them if there is no other option in order to keep everyone safe and get veterinary help.

A suitably sized pet carrier that your pet is used to sitting or travelling in is the safest way to transport them to the vet.

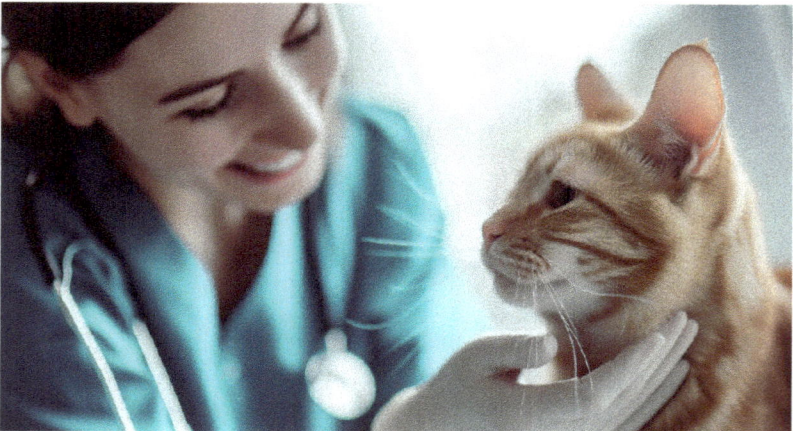

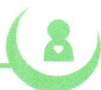

Put a favourite toy or blanket in the carrier with them as familiar objects will reduce the amount of stress that they are experience.

It is critically important to continually reassure your pet as stress can make symptoms worse.

Keep them calm and warm. Ideally, they should not have anything to eat or drink as they may require an operation. However, if they are dehydrated, or they could be waiting a considerable time for help, you should give them small sips of water. Ideally check with your Vet first.

If it is a life-threatening emergency – tell the Vet immediately.

Cat's name, breed, gender and date of birth

IS THE CASUALTY:

- **CONSCIOUS?**

- **UNCONSCIOUS AND BREATHING?**

- **NOT BREATHING?**

When you get to the vet they will need the following information:
- Cat's name and date of birth, breed, gender and weight
- Micro-chipping details
- Vaccination information
- Insurance details
- Medical conditions
- Medication
- Previous medical history

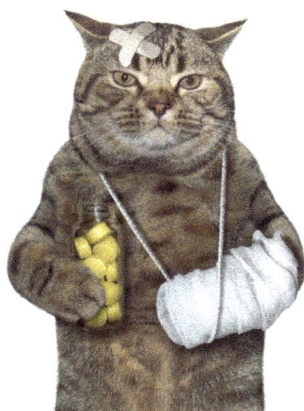

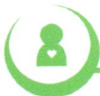

First Aid Kits

First Aid kits need to be easily accessible in case an emergency situation arises. The kit should be well organised, ideally in a bag with compartments to allow you to quickly grab what you need.

Whatever you have in your First Aid Kit, the most important thing is that it is good quality. Many kits tick the boxes in term of contents but are of such poor quality that should they need to use it, they would be of no use.

A First Aid kit designed for humans will be helpful in many medical emergencies, however additional aspects need to be considered for pets as they may need to be muzzled to prevent them biting you and they are also more likely to try and chew and remove any dressings that they may find irritating.

Your kit should contain as a minimum: a first aid book or instructions, and contents to treat: major and minor bleeding, burns, breaks and sprains.

A First Aid kit for humans should not contain medication. First Aid kits for a car should be in soft padded cases or secured within the car.

Always check your first aid kit and ensure everything remains in date and the packaging clean and in good condition. Out of date and damaged dressings may no longer be sterile and could cause infection.

Emergency Pet First Aid Book or access to an online pet first aid course

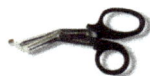

Tough cut scissors – strong enough to cut through clothes. Sharp ones to cut away fur and blunt ended ones to minimise the risk of injury

Face shield to protect yourself when doing animal CPR

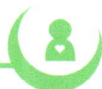

Gloves

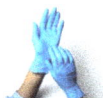

Sterile gauze and saline to clean a wound

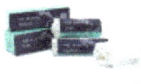

Gauze wound dressings of various sizes

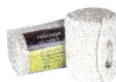

Micropore tape to secure dressings and also useful for labelling things

A couple of calico triangular bandages (ensure they are calico not a cheap version made of paper) these are some of the most useful things in your kit. Ideal, sterile, non-fluffy material to stop bleeding and can also be useful to make an improvised muzzle

Sterile saline vial – for irrigating a wound, or washing grit from an eye

Crepe bandage – for supporting a sprain or strain and could also be used for an improvised muzzle

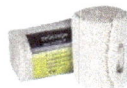

Self-adhesive bandage that will stick to itself without tape or pins

Cotton wool wadding to pad over the top of the sterile gauze, or padding around claws if you are bandaging.

Additional useful contents

Burn gel or a burns dressing – to apply to a burn after cooling

Instant ice pack to reduce swelling – at home you can use a bag of frozen peas – **Ensure it is wrapped in a cloth** as it can cause ice burns

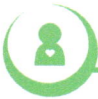

Instant heat pack to warm a pet suffering from hypothermia.

A foil blanket to keep the casualty warm, crucially important in helping to prevent them going into shock. They should ideally be insulated from the ground and have this wrapped round them to retain their body heat.

Sterile tweezers – for removing small splinters or thorns, that can easily be grasped and pulled out in the same direction that they went in (nothing else should ever be removed from a wound unless by a Vet)
Elizabethan Collar to prevent

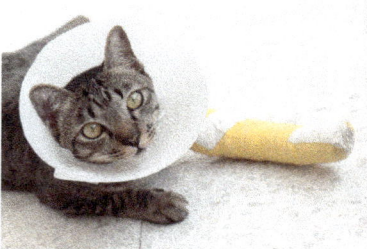

them from removing dressings and biting wounds.

A rectal thermometer and lubrication jelly
Blankets and newspaper to maintain hygiene and absorb any bodily fluids

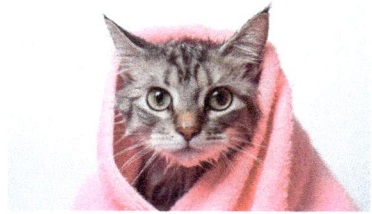

Small torch

Syringes – useful for irrigating a wound or giving medication

Cat booties for a paw injury

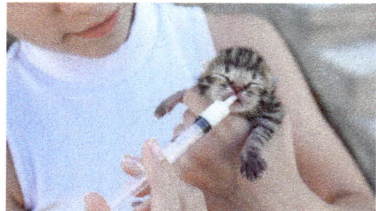

Pet dehydration medication, ask advice from your Vet

Antibiotic ointment – prescribed by your Vet

Antihistamine medication – prescribed by your Vet

NEVER GIVE HUMAN MEDICATION TO YOUR CAT unless specifically instructed to by the Vet

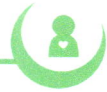

How to muzzle a cat

Even if it is your pet, if a cat is frightened and in pain, they are quite likely to bite.

Human safety always comes first. However, you should never muzzle an animal that is overheated (as they will need to pant to cool) or that is having difficulty breathing or is likely to vomit.

The following information shows you step by step how to create a comfortable and safe improvised muzzle for your pet.

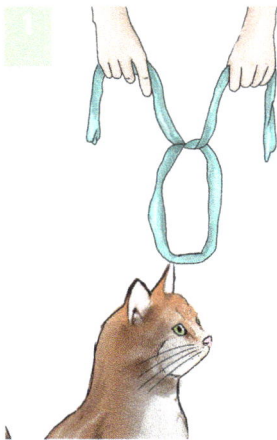

Use a bandage, scarf, tie or other soft material

• Make a loop in the material

• Gently and carefully restrain your pet

• Stand behind them and swiftly and calmly secure the loop over their snout (muzzle)

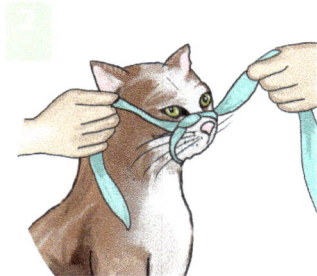

With a single knot on the top of their nose, secure the material around their snout to keep their mouth closed.

• Tie another knot under their chin and bring the ends back behind their ears.

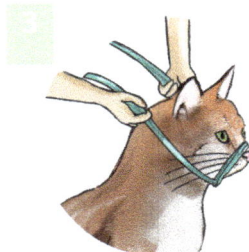

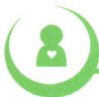

- Secure the ends with a slipknot or bow behind the animal's neck

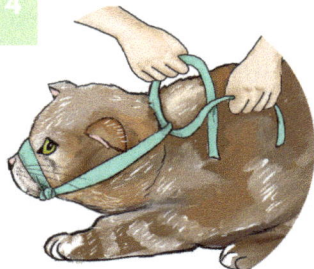

- Always have quick access to scissors to ensure you are able to swiftly release the muzzle should you need to do so.

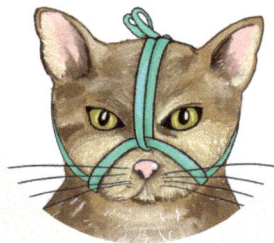

For a cat, as they have such short noses, you would then add in a further loop and pass it under the loop over the nose and tie it to the other end around the neck.

An alternative to muzzling:

You can also subdue a cat by gently dropping a towel on them, well above and behind them. Ensure you know the position of the cat as you drop the towel, to ensure you don't put your hands near their mouth.

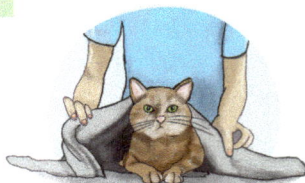

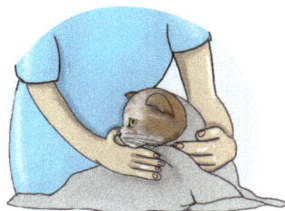

Grasp them by the scruff of their neck and wrap the towel around them completely encasing their paws, and just leaving their head exposed.

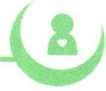

This should help you to be able to safely examine and treat them.

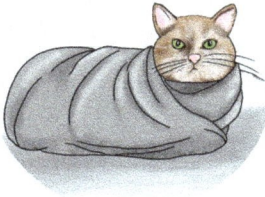

NEVER muzzle an animal that is having difficulty breathing, has a raised body temperature or is at risk of vomiting.

It is possible for an animal to bite even when muzzled in this way.

Be ready to release the muzzle if necessary. Do not put yourself at risk. If you are in danger of being bitten and are not confident using an improvised muzzle, phone the Vet and seek further advice.

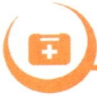

Primary Survey

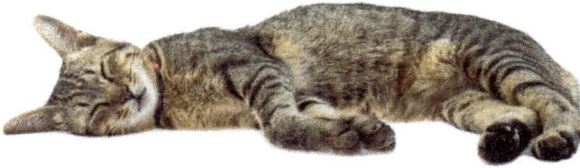

The Primary Survey is a fast and systematic way to find and treat any life-threatening conditions in order of priority:

Danger - Human safety always takes priority

Response - check to see if they are conscious

Airway - is their airway clear?

Breathing - are they breathing?

Circulation / CPR

DRABC – Action at an emergency

This section will take you through the actions required in a step-by-step guide for your quick reference in an emergency. We will cover this in more detail later to help you better understand the importance of each step.

Danger – Human safety always takes priority – always check it is safe for you and others

Phone the Vet as soon as possible and always take their advice.

Response – check to see if they are conscious

Approach from behind, initially touch with your foot.

If no response to a foot touch, use the back of your hand (less invasive than using your palm).

Touch or stroke to see if there is a response

Airway – is their airway clear?

Cautiously check in their mouth and tilt their head back to open

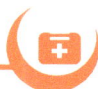

Breathing – are they breathing? – look down their body to see if they are breathing

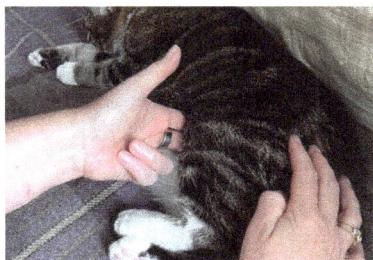

Circulation / CPR

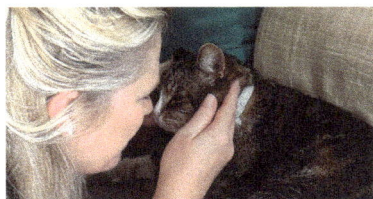

If they are unconscious and not breathing – give 30 chest compressions followed by 2 rescue breaths.

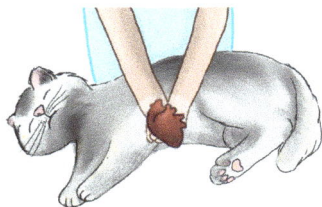

If there has been no response in 15 minutes it is extremely unlikely that they will recover.

Danger   **D**

Be aware of anything that could fall on you, be particularly careful on roads ensuring that traffic is aware there has been an accident and you are not putting yourself at risk.

Always check for electrical cables, broken glass, chemicals and make sure you do not put yourself at risk.

Approach all injured animals with caution and remain as calm as possible. Be prepared to muzzle them if necessary.

When administering to them it is best to be behind them, with their back to you if they are lying down, as they are less likely to bite from that angle.

If there is any danger – remove it. If the animal is being electrocuted, the electricity should be turned off at the mains before they are touched, otherwise you could be electrocuted as well.

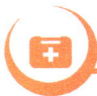

USE FACE SHIELD IF YOU ARE GIVING CPR

WEAR GLOVES WHEN DEALING WITH BLEEDING

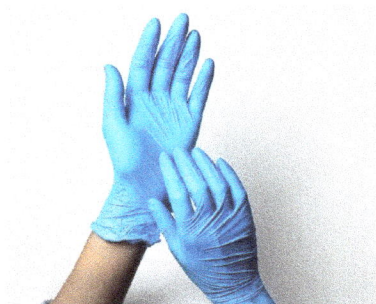

Make sure that everyone is safe. You are of no help to anyone if you become an additional casualty.

- **Be very aware of potential Danger**

- **If necessary, carefully remove the injured animal to safety. Ideally use an improvise stretcher such as a car parcel shelf and move them as little as possible.**

- **Be aware that animals that are scared and in pain are far more likely to bite – stand behind them to treat them and use a muzzle if necessary.**

Response — R

Never put yourself at risk. Establish as quickly as possible whether or not they are conscious:

Approach cautiously from behind. Initially touch them gently with your foot.

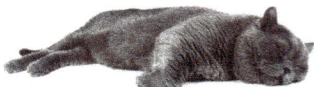

If there is no response when you touch with your foot, stroke them with the back of your hand.

If they are floppy and there is no response: Put them on a hard, level surface on their side

Quickly check if they are still alive – Check for breathing and put into the recovery position or start CPR accordingly.

Airway — A

When a cat is unconscious / unresponsive most of their muscles relax and go floppy.

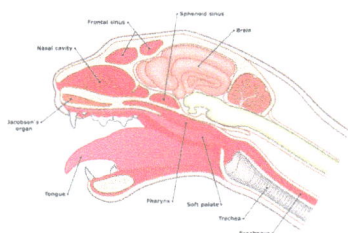

The tongue is a huge muscle attached to your bottom jaw and in a cat this rolls back and can block the airway. To open a cat's airway very carefully pull the tongue forward between the front teeth to clear it from the back of the throat. (Please note you would never do this with a human). Be especially careful that you do not get bitten

- It is also sensible to remove their collar and anything else that could cause any form of constriction and make it harder for them to breathe

- Pull their front legs forward so they are not resting on their chest

- If you are aware of vomit or excessive amounts of saliva in their throat, you should hold them upside down to allow this to drain

- With extreme caution (do not risk being bitten) look down their throat to see if there is an obvious obstruction and if there is, very carefully try and remove it. The Heimlich manoeuvre (animal abdominal thrust) is ideal to dislodge items in an animal's throat and this will be covered in the choking section

Breathing ──────────── **B**

To check for breathing; if possible, lie them on their side extend their head back and a little lower than the rest of their body, open their mouth and look at their chest movements, listen and feel to see if they are breathing.

If they are unresponsive and breathing normally keep them on their side with their head and neck extended slightly and their mouth open in an animal recovery position.

If the animal is unresponsive and not breathing normally you may wish to give them *artificial respiration*:

Circulation — C

The easiest way to check for cyanosis (whether they have reduced oxygen circulating in their blood) is to look at their mucous membranes in their gums or around their eyes. If these have a blue tinge rather than being red, they are low on oxygen.

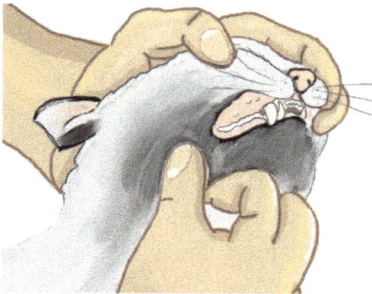

Unresponsive and Breathing

- If you are sure that they are breathing, keep them on their side, extend their head back to open their airway.

- Keep checking their pulse and breathing and call the Vet immediately.

- They will advise you the best way to move them.

- Be prepared to start CPR if they stop breathing.

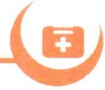

Recovery Position

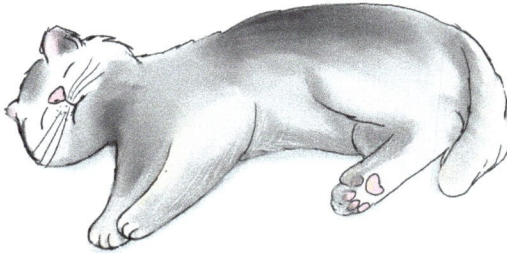

If you are sure that they are **unresponsive and breathing**, the best position to help them maintain an open airway is to put them into the recovery position, **on their side.** Extend their head back slightly to keep the tongue forward off the back of their throat and their airway clear.

Keep checking that they are breathing feeling their breath using the back of your hand in front of their mouth or by holding a wisp of fur in front of their nostrils to see if it moves as they exhale. Keep checking their pulse.

If you are concerned that they may be going into shock raise their hind quarters slightly raised and supported so that their body remains straight gravity encourages the tongue to flop forward and the contents of the stomach to drain out, so as to keep the airway clear and allow the animal to keep breathing.

Once in the Recovery position: keep checking that they are breathing feeling their breath using the back of your hand in front of their mouth or by holding a wisp of fur in front of their nostrils to see if it moves as they exhale.

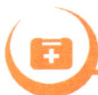

Resuscitation: CPR (Cardio Pulmonary Resuscitation)

When you are resuscitating, you are being a life support machine

When you push on their chest – you are being their heart

When you breathe into them – you are being their lungs

You are keeping their heart and brain full of oxygenated blood and keeping them alive so that when you get them to the Vet there is a chance of bringing them back to life.

Check for Danger, Check for Response, Open the Airway and check for Breathing

Unconscious and not breathing
Phone the Vet

Clear their airway; extend their neck back, pull their tongue forward and check to see if there is any obvious obstruction.

• Ideally lie your pet on their side – check for a pulse

Use a Face Shield to protect yourself

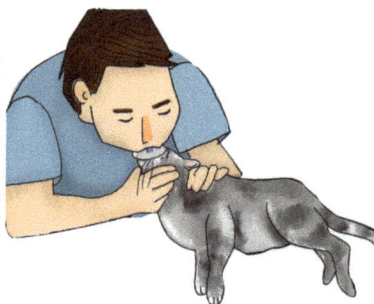

If your pet does not start breathing, **then CPR will give them the best chance.**

Chest compressions

CPR should only ever be performed on an animal that is unconscious and not breathing

Always gain permission before performing CPR on someone else's cat.

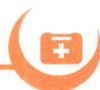

- If they are unconscious and not breathing, push on the chest just behind the front legs at a rate of about 100 to 120 times per minute

- Push down approximately a quarter to a third of their chest depth

- Give two breaths into the nose for every 30 compressions of the chest

- Keep going until at the veterinary practice – 30 compressions to 2 breaths - 30:2 - 30:2 - 30:2....

- If there are two people rotate every 2 minutes to minimise fatigue

- Realistically if your pet does not recover within an absolute maximum of 20 minutes it is very unlikely they will do so. (The Blue Cross state that if they haven't recovered within 3 minutes then recovery is incredibly unlikely)

For most cats: lie them on their side. Place the heel of one hand in the centre of their chest above where you can normally feel their heartbeat.

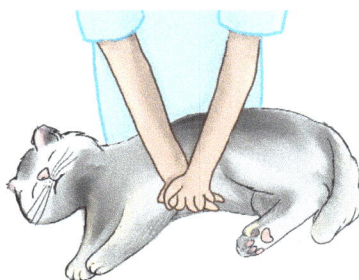

Resuscitation – What exactly are you doing?

When you are resuscitating, you are being a life support machine.

When you push on their chest – you are being their heart and when you breathe into them – you are being their lungs. You are keeping their heart and brain full of oxygenated blood and keeping them alive so that when you get them to the Vet there is a chance of bringing them back to life.

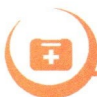

Choking

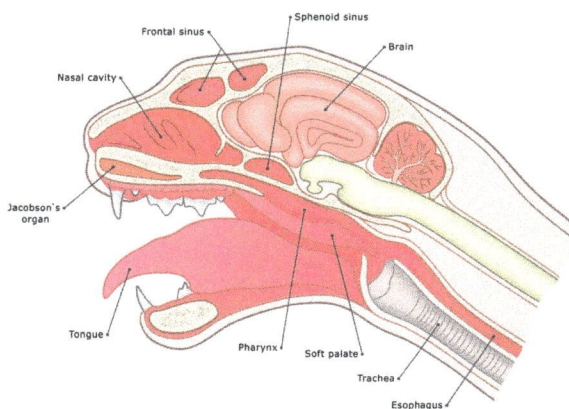

Choking occurs when something gets stuck in the back of the throat and blocks the airway. When the airway is partially blocked the animal may start retching, pacing back and forth and pawing at their mouth. If their airway becomes totally blocked they may be unable to make any sound at all.

Your pet may show clear signs of distress and paw at their mouth, gag or retch and drool, they are also likely to panic and may become wheezy. If they are struggling to breathe, they may appear to cough, struggle breathing and their mucous membranes may start turning blue. If untreated they will collapse and die.

Cats can choke on anything such as small balls, bones, socks, rubbish and children's toys. Choking is frightening and occasionally fatal.

Never delay getting Veterinary help and advice. Phone the Vet as soon as possible

How to recognise that they are choking – a choking cat may retch, pace or paw at its mouth.

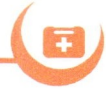

- **E**xtremely carefully look in their mouth, ideally with someone else helping. DO NOT GET BITTEN. Do not finger sweep of probe blindly to remove an obstruction as you will make things worse.

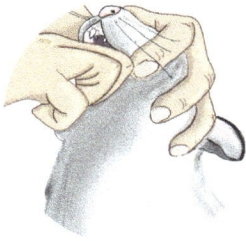

- If you can see something obvious, remove it with tweezers or forceps.

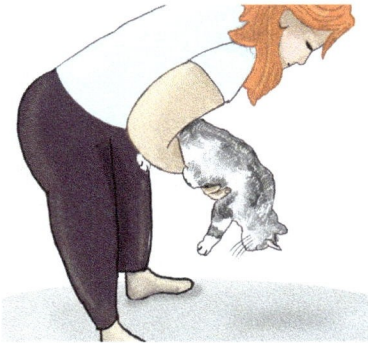

- Hold them upside down by their thighs and gently shake them to try and release the obstruction (please see picture above)

- If re-positioning them hasn't helped, you will need to do an abdominal thrust (Heimlich Manoeuvre):

- Stand behind your pet and reach over their back.

- Make a fist with one hand and place it under their abdomen, place the other hand over the fist and pull upwards and forwards under your pet's stomach.

- Repeat up to 5 times

- If your pet stops breathing you may need to be ready to help with rescue breathing and CPR

- If re-positioning them hasn't helped, you will need to do an abdominal thrust (Heimlich Manoeuvre):

- **Stand behind your pet and reach over their back.**

- Make a fist with one hand and place it under their abdomen, place the other hand over the fist and pull upwards and forwards under your pet's stomach.

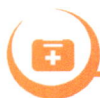

- Repeat up to 5 times

- If your pet stops breathing you may need to be ready to help with rescue breathing and CPR

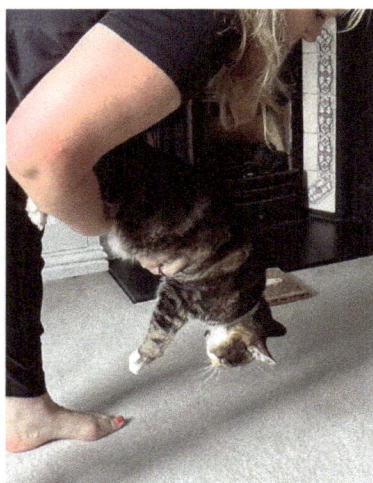

In most cases, getting rid of the choking obstruction allows the cat to begin breathing again on its own. Remember that as they are scared they are very likely to bite even when the object has been removed – they will also pick up on your panicked heart beat which will add to their fear and anxiety.

If your cat is unconscious and not breathing you may wish to begin CPR at approximately 120 chest compressions per minute, 30 compressions to 2 breaths and continue these until at the veterinary practice.

Whether the item is dislodged or not, it is essential that the animal is thoroughly checked by a Vet as there may be damage to the inside of the mouth or throat once the object is removed, or damage to their ribs or internal organs if you have attempted a Heimlich Manoeuvre.

Trauma to the inside of the mouth or throat can take many days to heal, and can also make it hard or painful for the cat to eat his regular food. Making the normal diet soft by running it through the blender with warm water may help. Your vet may dispense pain relief to help during the recovery period.

Suffocation and strangulation has similar symptoms to choking but you are likely to be able to

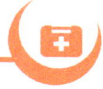

spot the cause relatively easily. Strangulation can be caused by a cable, string or other item wrapped around the neck, carefully use a pair of scissors to cut the object. Suffocation is most commonly caused by plastic bags, if possible carefully remove and treat as for unconscious not breathing.

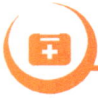

Drowning

NEVER risk your life for a drowning pet – do not go into water to rescue your pet.

Your cat may be able to swim. However, if they become trapped or tired it is still possible for them to drown.

If you find your pet unconscious in water –

- Check the mucous membranes for a grey or bluish discolouration which would mean that they are cyanosed.

- Check for breathing

- If you are able to, hold your pet upside down and gently shake them.

- Alternatively put them onto their right hand side with their head lower than their body.

- Locate the last ribs and push into the dent beside these in an upward motion towards their head to try and force out any water.

- Repeat this 4 or 5 times and continue for about a minute

- If they do not begin to come round or start breathing and there is no pulse – Start rescue breaths and then if appropriate: CPR.

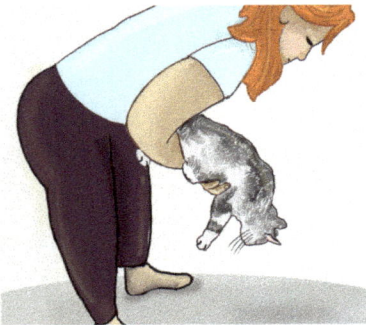

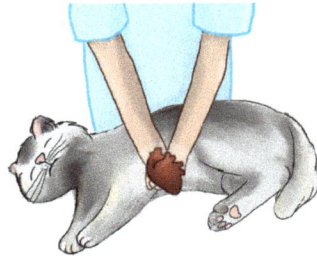

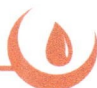

Wounds and Bleeding

WEAR GLOVES WHEN DEALING WITH BLEEDING

Always dispose of soiled dressings in a yellow incinerator bag.

If your pet is bleeding the priority is to stop the blood coming out!

It is not a priority to clean the wound

If the wound is deep or bleeding profusely, do not attempt to clean it as this should be done by the Vet in a clinical environment. Ideally all wounds should be seen by a Vet, however if the wound is minor and you are not planning to get it seen by a vet, then this should be carefully cleaned before it is dressed

You may need to carefully trim your pet's fur around the wound so that you can properly see the extent of the damage. Ideally use curved scissors to do this to avoid accidentally cutting their skin.

A wound can be cleaned using saline or clean water. For very dirty wounds you may wish to use an approved animal antiseptic – although a dirty wound should always be seen and treated by a vet.

Do not use Hydrogen Peroxide as this can damage the edges of the wound and it could take longer to heal.

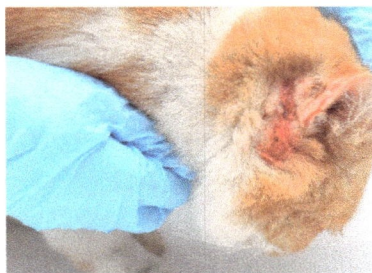

All bite wounds should be seen by a Vet so they can properly assess the extent of the damage and your pet is likely to need antibiotics

Types of bleeding

Arterial bleeding

An arterial bleed is expelled under pressure from the heart and is bright red and frothy. An animal with an arterial bleed can lose blood very fast and quickly go into shock. It is vitally important to apply pressure fast to stop the bleeding.

Venous bleeding

Venous blood is darker than arterial blood and pours rather than spurts. Venous bleeding is easier to control than arterial bleeding.

Internal bleeding

It is also possible that your pet could be bleeding internally, and this can be recognised by your pet becoming cold, restless, pale gums, having a fast heartbeat and shallow breathing, little or no urine, dark concentrated urine or blood in the urine. Lethargic and floppy or visible blood coming from any of their orifices. If you suspect internal bleeding it is vitally important that you get veterinary help fast

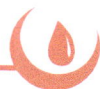

Treatment of bleeding

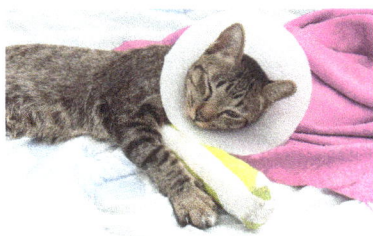

- If you are applying a bandage to your pet it is vitally important that you do not put it on too tight.

- Never bandage or try to splint a limb that you think is broken as you will make things worse. Always phone the Vet and adhere to their advice.

- If you are bandaging the lower limb, you should cover the foot. But you must ensure that you check the paw regularly to ensure that it is not swelling. If you have any concerns you must call the Vet.

- If you are applying a bandage at home, it should be checked by a Vet as soon as possible.

- Never leave a bandage on for longer than 24 hours unless applied by a Vet.

- Avoid the bandage getting wet as this will make it tighter and can lead to the wound becoming infected. Avoid taking your cat out in wet conditions. Your Vet will often be able to provide used IV fluid bags to try and protect the bandage from getting wet

Cover the cleaned wound with a sterile dressing

Clean the wound. Use a sterile non-adherent dressing to cover the cleaned wound.

Protect their claws by placing cotton wool between each toe

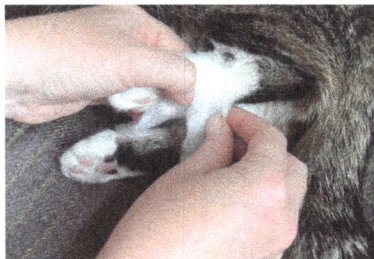

Carefully place small pieces of cotton wool between each claw, including the thumb and dew claw.

Wrap cushioning bandage from paw to the next joint

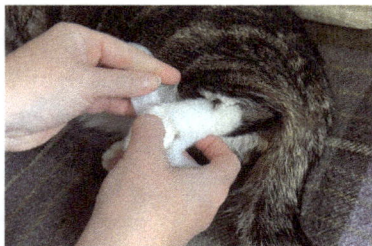

Starting at the paw cover with soft band (cushioning lightweight cotton wool type bandage)

Bandage from the foot to the next joint

Apply a layer of cohesive bandage over the top

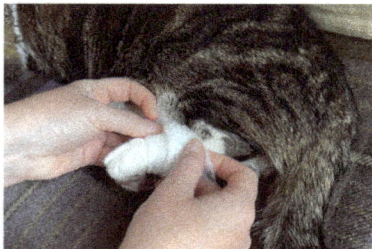

Cover the entire bandage with Vetwrap

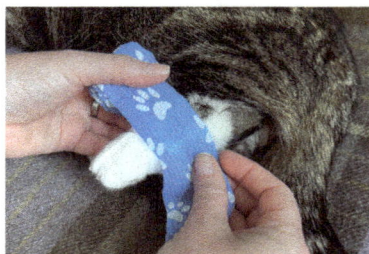

Cover the entire bandage with a Vetwrap pet bandage which is a cohesive bandage that sticks to itself as you bandage and is stronger than human bandages – ensure you are not putting it on too tight.

Start by going under the paw and take the bandage all the way up to the next joint.

Ensure the bandage is firm, but not too tight.

Continually observe to ensure their paw does not start to swell.

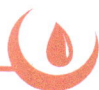

If worried remove the bandage immediately

- **Do not leave the bandage on for more than 24 hours**

- **Get veterinary advice as soon as possible**

- **Do not allow the bandage to get wet as it will become tighter and the wound is more likely to become infected. (Veterinary Practices often give IV bags to cover bandages)**

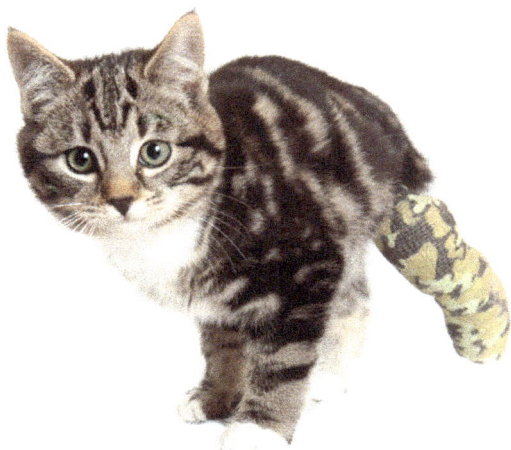

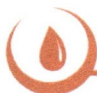

Embedded objects

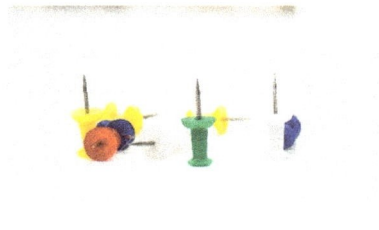

Pad above the object using rolled bandages or a rolled donut ring to allow you to bandage over the object to prevent it getting knocked on the way to the Vet

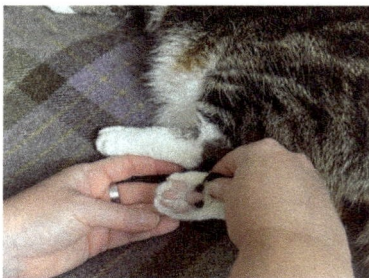

Do not remove the embedded object from the wound, as it will have damaged on the way in and will damage again on the way out! It may also be stemming any bleeding.

Apply pressure without pushing on the embedded object

Use a rolled cloth or triangular bandage to make a donut ring and then apply pressure over the wound without pushing the object further in. Call the Vet.

Either use 2 rolled bandages either side of the embedded object or a triangular bandage rolled into a donut ring.

What if there is glass in the wound?

If you suspect that there is a glass in the wound, your pet may need an x-ray.

Never remove anything embedded in a wound, with the exception of a small splinter that is clearly visible and easy to remove. If the splinter is on a joint it should only be removed by a vet as it is possible that the joint capsule may have been damaged and this could lead to infection.

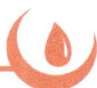

Splinters

• Clean the wound with warm soapy water

• Use a pair of clean tweezers, grip the splinter close to the skin and gently pull the splinter out at the same angle as it appears to have entered.

• Gently squeeze around the wound to encourage a little bleeding and ensure that there is nothing else remaining in the wound. Clean the wound once more and then cover with a breathable sterile dressing.

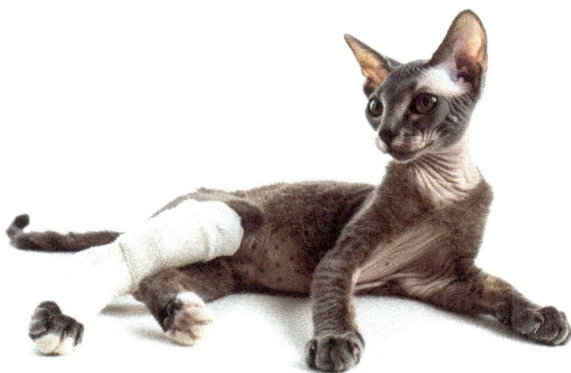

Nosebleeds

Animals get nose bleeds due to injury, foreign bodies, tumours, infections, poisoning or high blood pressure.

The majority of time it is just a minor injury and applying pressure and cooling them will help.

However, if the bleeding lasts longer than 15 minutes or the bleeding is heavy you should contact your Vet straight away.

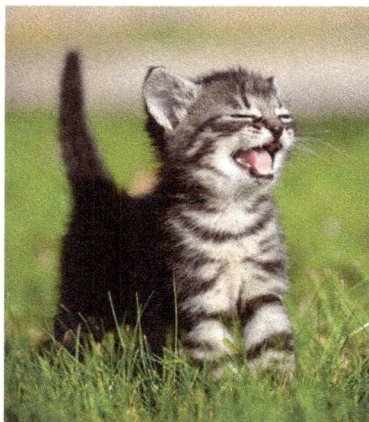

How to treat a nosebleed

- Ideally wear gloves

- Grab something to catch the blood

- Cool the nose with a cool pack or bag of frozen peas wrapped in a cloth

- Apply pressure for at least 10 minutes,

- Release pressure slightly and if it starts to bleed again, hold for a bit longer

IF BLEEDING IS EXTREMELY HEAVY OR CONTINUES FOR MORE THAN 15 MINUTES CONTACT YOUR VET ASAP

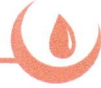

Bite wounds

Bite wounds can be extremely distressing for both the cat and their owner. Stop the bleeding by applying pressure to the wound with a clean cloth. Get them to the Vet as soon as possible.

If possible, swap details with the owner of the other cat.

Stop the bleeding and get the wound seen by a Vet

A bite wound should always be cleaned properly by a Vet. The wound may penetrate further than you can easily see, and bite wounds nearly always require antibiotics as otherwise they are very likely to become infected.

WEAR GLOVES WHEN DEALING WITH BLEEDING

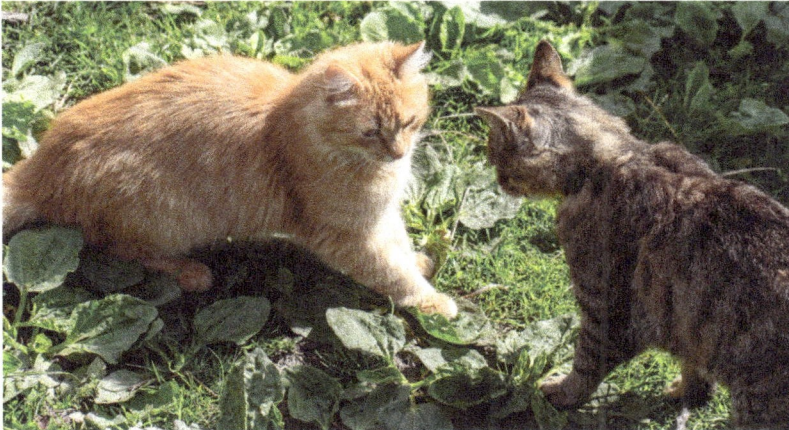

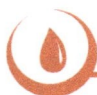

Eye Injuries

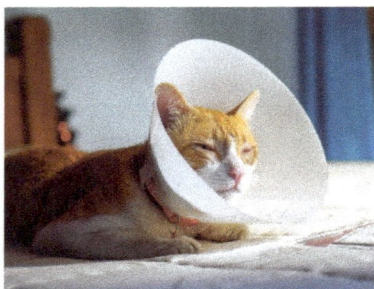

Eye injuries can be very unpleasant and painful.

Should the eye have come out of its socket or be bulging; it is important to prevent the eye from drying out and to reduce the risk of further damage and infection.

- Apply a dressing soaked in sterile saline solution.

- Prevent the animal from rubbing or scratching the eye (an Elizabethan collar is ideal for this) and call the vet.

- The dressing will need to remain wet whilst in transit to the Vet, so continually re-moisten the dressing with saline solution.

Chemicals in the Eye

If your pet gets chemicals in their eye, wash the eye immediately with cold water or a saline eye wash and transport to the nearest vet.

- Wear gloves.

- Rinse the eye with cool running water for at least 10 minutes, but ideally longer, . (most easily done using an eyes wash dispenser or alternatively a sports drinking bottle can be helpful)

- Cover the affected eye with a non-fluffy pad if necessary.

- Call the vet and arrange to have the pet transferred as soon as possible

- Take the bottle of chemical with you or take a photo of the label as this will be helpful to the Vet.

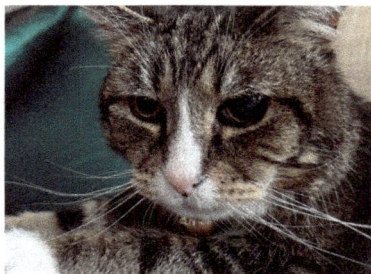

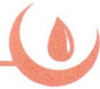

Shock

- Shock is 'a lack of oxygen to the tissues of the body, usually caused by a fall in blood volume or blood pressure.'

- Shock occurs as a result of the body's circulatory system failing to work properly, which means that the tissues and organs of the body, including the heart and the brain, struggle to get sufficient oxygen. The body's response to this is to shut down the circulation to the skin, the heart speeds up as it tries to get sufficient blood supply and oxygen around the body and blood supply is drawn away from the gut to prioritise vital organs; which causes the animal to feel sick and thirsty and can lead to collapse.

- Shock results from major drop in blood pressure and is serious.

The most common types of shock are:

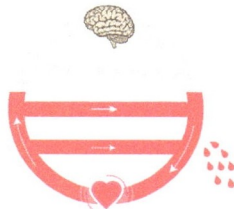

- Hypovolaemic – The body loses fluid, such as with major bleeds (internal and external), burns, diarrhoea and vomiting

- Cardiogenic – Heart attack – the heart is not pumping effectively

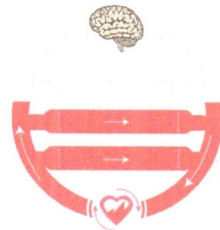

- Anaphylactic – The body reacts to something releasing large amounts of Histamine and other hormones – these dilate the blood vessels and cause them to leak fluid, causing swelling of the airways and leading to a triple whammy of shock.

- Extremes of temperature can also cause the body to go into Shock as can a major assault on the nervous system such as a spinal or brain injury.

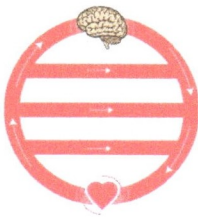

Normal Circulation   Hypovolaemic Shock   Anaphylactic Shock

Signs and Symptoms of shock

Initially:

- Rapid pulse
- Pale, cold and clammy

As shock develops:

- Grey-blue skin colour and blue tinge to the mucous membranes – cyanosed
- Weak and dizzy
- Nausea and vomiting
- Thirst
- Shallow, rapid breathing

As the brain is struggling for oxygen:

- May become restless and possibly aggressive
- Yawning and gasping for air
- Eventually they will lose consciousness and become unresponsive and finally stop breathing

Treatment for shock

Lie the animal on their side (ideally on their right hand side). Put a folded blanket under their lower back to raise it to encourage the blood more to their heart and brain.

Cover with a blanket to keep them warm

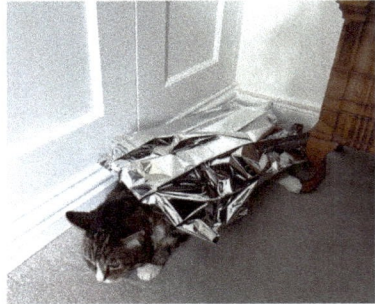

Shock is made worse when an animal is cold, anxious and in pain – reassuring them and keeping them warm can make a real difference.

Call the Vet immediately

Do not give them anything to eat or drink, as they may need an operation and it is safer to give someone a general anaesthetic when they have an empty stomach.

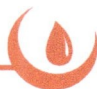

Clinical Shock

How to recognize and treat clinical shock

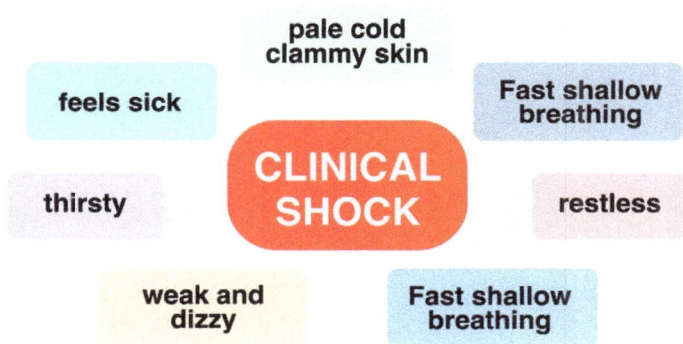

pale cold
clammy skin

feels sick

Fast shallow
breathing

**CLINICAL
SHOCK**

thirsty

restless

weak and
dizzy

Fast shallow
breathing

Road traffic accidents - how to help

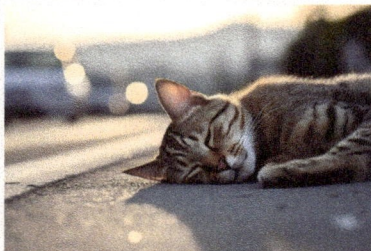

The following is a step by step approach as guidance should you be the first on scene at an accident:

Ensure your own safety, that of other humans and that of the injured animal

When approaching an accident scene the most important element is your safety. Make sure that all traffic has stopped and it is flagged up that there has been an accident otherwise there may be additional casualties. **Human safety and human casualties always take priority.**

Be aware of oncoming traffic to ensure that is not posing an additional danger. Note if there is any fuel spillage or potential fire risk – turn off car ignitions if possible. Put on hazard lights and encourage other cars to do the same.

Stay as calm as you can

• Stress and panic will make things worse for the injured animal.

• Try and reassure them

• Keep them warm and dry

Phone your Vet or the nearest veterinary surgery

The vet will want to know:

• what has happened?

• if your pet is conscious or unconscious ?

• are they bleeding?

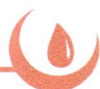

- where are they injured?

- where is the animal now and do you need to move them to allow traffic to begin moving again?

The Vet is likely to give you advice as to how to stabilize particular injuries and the best way to move the animal.

Consider muzzling your pet if there is a risk of you being bitten

Be aware that injured animals will be scared and in pain. Cats in pain and frightened are likely to bite, even if they know and love you, so an emergency muzzle can be made with some bandage or tape to loop over the cat's nose before **transporting or handling, or by wrapping them in a blanket or towel.**

Only use a muzzle IF the animal is not having breathing difficulties and is not at risk of vomiting.

Keep the injured animal warm

- Keep your cat warm by wrapping them in a blanket, coat or foil blanket

- Keep the nose and mouth exposed

- Carefully transport them directly to your nearest vet

- If there is a risk of a spinal injury you should do your best to avoid twisting your cat when transferring them to your vehicle

- A car parcel shelf or covered board can make a useful improvised stretcher

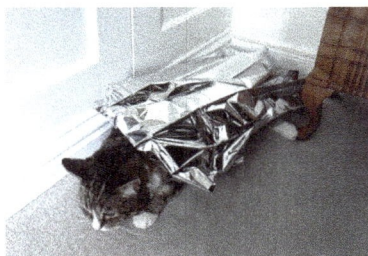

If your cat is having difficulty breathing

- If your cat is having trouble breathing; remove their collar, open their mouth and check for any obstructions

- If they are unconscious and breathing, place on their side in the recovery position

Treatment of wounds

Cover any wounds with a clean cloth and apply gentle pressure to stop bleeding.

Do not give food or drink to an injured animal in case they need an anaesthetic.

However, if there will be a delay getting veterinary treatment and your cat is distressed and dehydrated, on veterinary advice they may be given small amounts of water.

Do not give any medication unless directed to do so by the Vet.

Roll a dog or cat onto an improvised stretcher to transport them - avoid twisting their spine

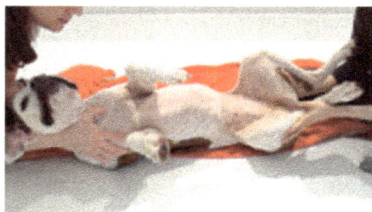

Avoid them twisting their spine. Everyone on the road should have a suitably stocked First Aid kit and know how to use its contents. Most of the contents of a human first aid kit can be useful to a cat in a medical emergency. Never give any human medication to a cat without Veterinary instructions to do so.

Support their head and neck and carefully roll them ideally onto a stiff board, car parcel shelf, or blanket to transfer them into the car.

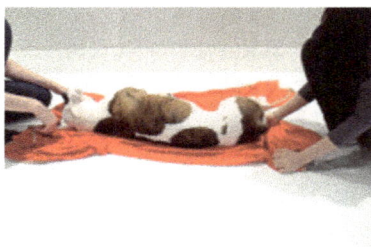

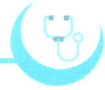

Allergic reaction

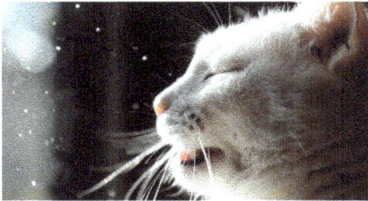

Allergic reactions occur because the body's immune system reacts inappropriately in response to the presence of a substance that it wrongly perceives as a threat. In order to develop an allergic response, the body has to be exposed to something in order to trigger the immune response – this can be touched, inhaled, swallowed or injected – during a routine vaccination or by an insect sting.

The body reacts to Histamine

The body doesn't react to the irritant directly but reacts to the histamine released by cells damaged through the immune response on subsequent exposure.

Pets can have an allergic reaction to all sorts of things; from bites and stings to grass, food or anything a human can react to.

They may be biting or licking the affected area

When you observe the area, it may be swollen, red and have visible allergic hives (raised red patches).

If they are having a minor skin allergy washing the area in cool water may help. Your vet will be able to prescribe an oral antihistamine if necessary.

It is also possible for your pet to have a life-threatening **anaphylactic reaction.** Diagnosed by some of the following signs and symptoms:

- Pain, itching, swelling and redness of the affected area

- Swelling of the face and neck

- Raised hives spreading over the body, face and neck

- Vomiting and diarrhoea

- Difficulty breathing

- Shock, collapse and unconsciousness

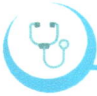

This is a serious medical emergency for your pet and they will need veterinary help extremely fast. Transport them to the Vet in the pet recovery position with their lower back slightly higher than the rest of the body (pad underneath their (pad underneath their body to keep their back straight) If they lose consciousness and stop breathing you may wish to start CPR.

If the reaction is caused by a bee sting and the sting is still visible – it should be scraped out using a credit card or thumbnail, but not removed with tweezers as this would squeeze more venom into the wound.

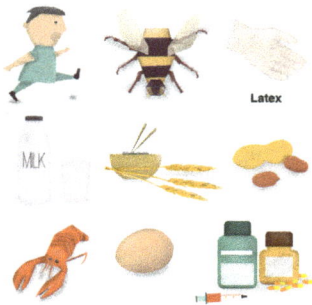

Your pet can develop a reaction to any foods and it can be very difficult to work out which one is the culprit.

Do not smoke around your pet and be careful which chemical cleaning products you use around your house.

If you see the animal begin to develop breathing problems and swelling around their throat, get Veterinary advice immediately.

How to treat Anaphylaxis and acute allergic reaction

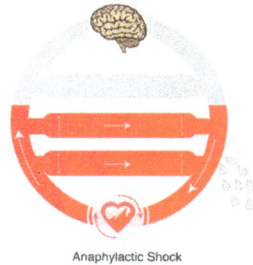

Anaphylactic Shock

Avoid allergens where possible

The key advice is to avoid any known allergens if at all possible.

Antihistamine can help mild allergic reactions

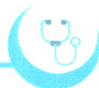

If an animal is having a mild allergic reaction, your Vet may prescribe an antihistamine tablet or syrup and this can be very effective. However, the medication will take at least 15 minutes to work. If you are concerned that the reaction could be systemic (all over) and life threatening, phone your Vet immediately.

Get Veterinary help fast

Your Vet is likely to give Adrenaline. Adrenaline (also known as epinephrine) acts quickly to constrict blood vessels, relax smooth muscles in the lungs to improve breathing, stimulate the heartbeat and helps to reduce swelling.

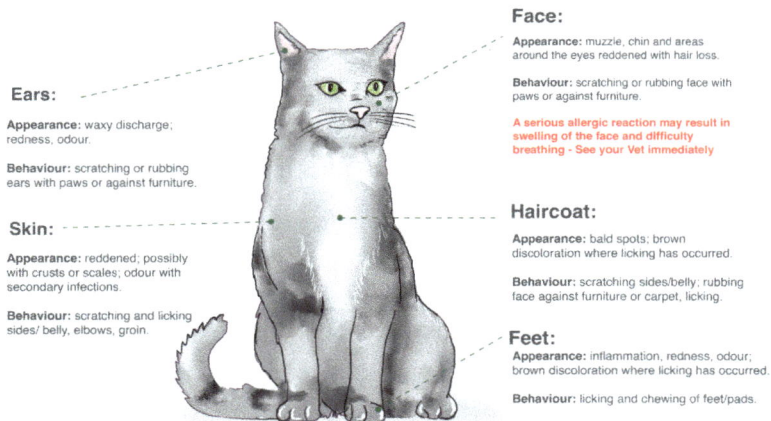

Ears:

Appearance: waxy discharge; redness, odour.

Behaviour: scratching or rubbing ears with paws or against furniture.

Skin:

Appearance: reddened; possibly with crusts or scales; odour with secondary infections.

Behaviour: scratching and licking sides/ belly, elbows, groin.

Face:

Appearance: muzzle, chin and areas around the eyes reddened with hair loss.

Behaviour: scratching or rubbing face with paws or against furniture.

A serious allergic reaction may result in swelling of the face and difficulty breathing - See your Vet immediately

Haircoat:

Appearance: bald spots; brown discoloration where licking has occurred.

Behaviour: scratching sides/belly; rubbing face against furniture or carpet, licking.

Feet:

Appearance: inflammation, redness, odour; brown discoloration where licking has occurred.

Behaviour: licking and chewing of feet/pads.

49

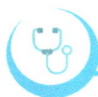

Bites and Stings

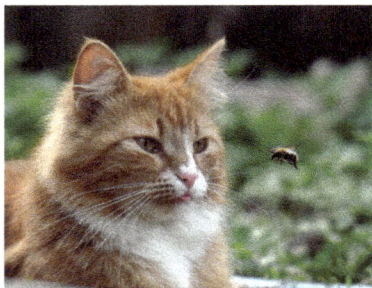

Bee and wasp stings

- Always protect yourself and ensure your own safety first.

- If your pet has been stung by a bee and the sting is visible, scape it out with your thumbnail or a credit card (a wasp does not leave a stinger behind). Applying a wrapped ice pack may help to soothe the sting and reduce inflammation. If the sting is in the mouth or throat, contact the vet as the sting may cause swelling which will interfere with breathing.

- If your pet appears to be having an allergic reaction you will need Veterinary help immediately.

- Wasps and other stinging insects do not leave the sting behind in the wound.

- If your pet has a local reaction, a wrapped ice pack applied to the area can quickly help to reduce the swelling.

- If your pet shows any signs of a systemic reaction or of anaphylactic shock, call your vet immediately as this is a life-threatening emergency.

Tick bites

Ticks are egg-shaped spider like creatures that are common in parks, woodland, grassland and heath areas. They are now present in most parks and it is important to check your cat for these following every walk.

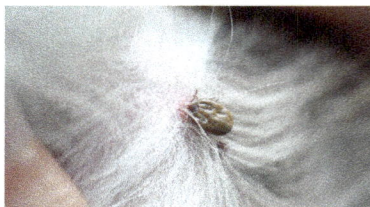

Ticks carry some serious diseases, so it's important to remove any that attach themselves to your cat. This is not easy, as you need to be careful not to squeeze the

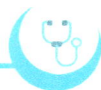

tick's body, or allow its head to get stuck inside your cat as residual bits of tick can lead to infection. Pet shops sell specific tick-removal devices which can make this process easier. Ask your vet for advice as there is also specific tick treatment available for ticks.

Lyme disease

Lyme disease is a serious illness carried by Ticks and it affects humans too. Visit your doctor if you experience flu like symptoms or extreme lethargy and let your doctor know that you have a pet and ask that they test you for Lyme's disease. You should get your pet tested at the Vet too.

Some people find that they develop a skin reaction around the site of the tick bite, and this is an obvious sign of Lyme disease – however a third of people can be infected with Lyme Disease without having a rash. The size of the rash can vary significantly, and it may expand over several days or weeks. Typically, it's around 15cm (6 inches) across, but it can be much larger or smaller than this. Some people may develop several rashes in different parts of their body.

Never burn the tick off or try and use chemicals to kill it. Keep the tick in a container to show to the vet so they can ensure has been removed entirely.

Flea bites

Flea bites are annoying and itchy for most cats, but if your cat is allergic to them then they can cause real discomfort and severe scratching, which can become infected.

If your pet has a large infestation of fleas, this can cause them to become anaemic.

Flea Allergy Dermatitis (FAD) is incredibly common and is sensitivity to flea saliva.

The saliva of just one or two fleas can cause them to become itchy and uncomfortable for many weeks, long past the death of the original fleas.

Fleas can be treated with many different over the counter remedies. Alternatively ask your Vet or Grooming Parlour for recommendations.

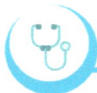

Snake Bites

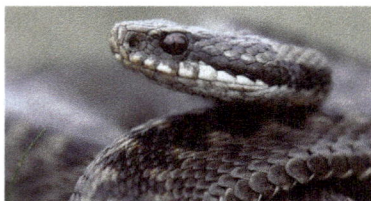

Snakes tend to bite if threatened and this means that cats are more likely to be bitten than humans.

The adder is the only poisonous snake in the wild in the UK, however some venomous exotic snakes are kept as pets. If you think your cat has been bitten by an adder, call your vet straight away as cats are likely to survive adder bites if they are treated quickly.

Recognising a snake bite

- Local swelling that is often dark coloured and can become severe.

- You may be able to see 2 small puncture wounds in the centre of the swelling.

- Bites most commonly occur on a cat's legs or face.

- Signs of pain or nervousness

- Pale mucous membranes (gums), bruising, salivation/dribbling, vomiting, diarrhoea, dehydration, restlessness, drowsiness and lethargy

- Animal may collapse, have blood clotting problems, tremors or convulsions

- Bites on or around the face can lead to swelling of the face and muzzle, resulting in breathing difficulties

Seek veterinary attention

Seek veterinary attention quickly if your cat is bitten. Carry your cat (rather than allow them to walk) to try and prevent the spread of venom around their body. Apply a wrapped ice pack to help control the swelling and keep your cat calm and warm as you transport them to the vet.

If possible, keep the wound below the level of the heart
If they show signs of anaphylaxis treat appropriately

If they stop breathing – start CPR

NEVER use a tourniquet as this will cut off the blood supply to the whole limb and is likely to make things worse.

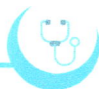

Tip – If you have seen the snake it is really helpful to try and remember its markings and head shape to describe to the medical professionals.

Animal bites

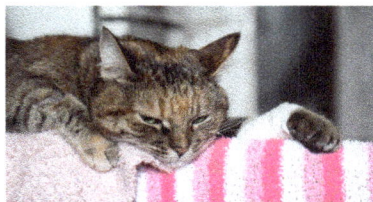

Bites from cats and other animals can be jagged and frequently get infected. Even if an animal bite has just punctured the skin, it is important to wash the wound really well and look out for any signs of infection. It is sensible to get any bite that has punctured the skin looked at by a Vet. Even a quite small looking wound can be deceptively large and there can be considerable damage underneath the skin and fur. Bites quickly get infected, they need to be thoroughly cleaned by a medical professional and Vet's usually prescribe antibiotics.

If the wound looks red and becomes inflamed, hot, or angry looking, it is getting infected they will definitely need antibiotics.

Treating the bite

The initial treatment for an animal bite is the same as for any other wound, except it is important to wash it immediately with clean water and antibacterial soap. The steps are as follows:

• Reassure your pet and phone the Vet. All bite wounds should be seen by a Vet asap.

• If the vet is unavailable – wash the wound thoroughly with clean water (and antibacterial soap depending on the location of the wound)

• stop any bleeding

• elevate the wound and apply pressure to stop bleeding

• Get to a Vet as soon as you can

Note : Outside the UK, if a human is bitten or licked in a wound, it is really important to get medical attention very fast and have anti-rabies medication. It is also important to ensure that they are covered for tetanus.

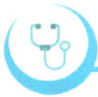

Burns

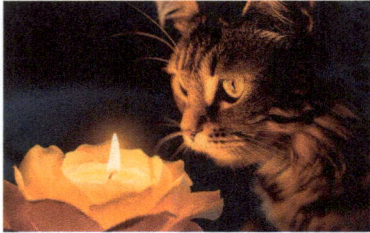

Safety first

If your cat is burnt, the priority is still to ensure your own safety and ensure that everyone is safe from further danger and then for minor burns cool the burn as quickly as possible.

Keep yourself safe, avoid getting burnt yourself – turn off power, extinguish flames – Avoid getting bitten – muzzle your pet if necessary.

Cool running water

• Run the burn under cool running water for at least ten minutes (ideally for 20), draining from the nearest exit point so that water is not running unnecessarily over your pet.

• Call the vet

Further treatment and advice

Keep your pet warm and do your best to avoid them going into shock

Avoid touching the burn and wear sterile gloves if at all possible

Do not apply any burns or creams

Never apply ice to a burn

Never burst blisters

This advice relates to First Aid for minor burns on animals; for more serious burns where the skin has become visibly blistered or damaged, you should get Veterinary advice immediately and do as instructed by them.

Size, Cause, Age, Location, Depth all affect how severely your pet is burned

Size – the larger the area involved, the more serious it is for your pet and the more likely they are to suffer from shock, due to the loss of fluid from the burn. Pain, stress and being cold will make

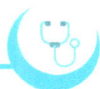

shock worse, so it is important to try and remain calm and keep the rest of your pet warm, whilst cooling the burn. Get veterinary advice quickly.

Cause – a burn can be caused by many different things

- Scalds are common injuries to pets caused by spills from hot liquids, such as kettles, saucepans full of hot water, hot drinks

- In a house fire the flames will burn the fur and skin, but animals can also gain burns to their airways from the heat contained in the air which, when breathed in, damages the delicate linings within the lungs. Smoke inhalation is also a concern and if they have been involved in a house fire your pet must always be checked by a Vet to prevent serious breathing problems.

- Electrical Injuries occur most commonly in the home if your pet chews an electrical flex. Always turn off the mains electricity before touching your pet as otherwise you will be electrocuted too.

- Chemical burns are most commonly caused by household cleaners and garden chemicals. De-icing products and rock salt in winter can also burn a cat's paws.

Age – burns are more serious in **kittens** than in older cats

Location – burns to the; paws, face, genitals, airways, or a burn that extends all the way around a limb, are particularly serious. Keep the burnt area under cool running water and contact the nearest vet immediately.

Depth – superficial, partial thickness or full thickness burns – The advice for First Aid treatment for animal burns relates to superficial burns – For more serious burns where the skin is visibly damaged, call the Vet and adhere to their advice.

Burns are serious.

Often pets have different depths of burn within a single injury.

Determine the depth of the burn:

- **Superficial burn** has just

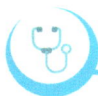

affected the top layer of skin, it is really painful and likely to blister

- *Partial thickness* burn is really painful. The burn has gone through both the first and second layer of skin

- *Full thickness burns* are often not as painful as the nerves have been very severely damaged too. This is the most severe sort of burn, the skin may appear pale, white or charred it will require extensive treatment and skin grafts.

Sunburn

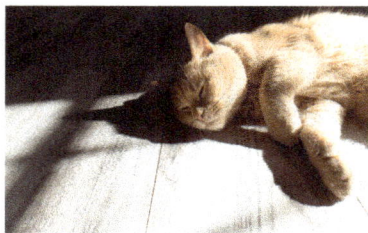

Prevent sunburn by avoiding the main heat of the day. Light coloured cats and those with very thin fur or hairless are particularly susceptible to sunburn and it may be sensible to apply a pet sun cream.

Remember that the pads of their feet can also get burnt on hot surfaces and tarmac and think carefully about taking them out in the midday sun.

Pet sunscreens are available – use a sunscreen designed for pets as it is likely that they will try and lick it off. If your pet does experience sunburn:

- Cool the area under a shower for at least 10 minutes (ideally a full 20 minutes), or apply repeated cool wet towels for 15 minutes.

- When completely cooled, apply neat Aloe Vera gel to the affected area, this will soothe, reduce swelling and promote healing.

- Give your pet plenty to drink and seek advice from your Vet.

Chemical burns

If the burn is caused by a *chemical*, run under cool running water for at least 20 minutes and be careful of the runoff as it could still be corrosive and hurt you. Look at the advice on the packaging and see if there

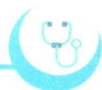

are any specific instructions. In winter, always inspect your cat's paws, rinse and wipe them to remove any residue of rock salt or de-icing products.

Caustic substances most commonly affect the feet and mouth/tongue (from licking to clean themselves).

• Don't get bitten. Muzzle your pet.

• Wear gloves and protect yourself from contamination.

• Open windows and doors to ensure the area is well ventilated.

• If the burn is from a dry chemical, brush away as much of the substance as possible. A pillowcase over the head would be useful to protect the mouth, nose and eyes from further contamination whilst brushing off.

• Rinse the contaminated area with large amounts of tepid (warm) flowing water, a shower is good for this. Wear gloves, safety glasses and mask to protect yourself

• If the chemical is in the pet's eyes, flush with clean water or sterile saline for 15-20 minutes.

• Do not put anything else on the burn

• NEVER apply ice to the burn.

• Carefully transport to the closest vet and take the chemical's container with you if possible.

Smoke inhalation

If your pet has been involved in a fire they should always be examined for smoke inhalation.

• Smoke and heat can damage the lining of the respiratory tract as can noxious fumes.

• Carbon monoxide competes with oxygen binding with the haemoglobin in the blood. This means that your pet does not have enough oxygen in their blood and this can be fatal.

Carefully transport the animal to the closest Vet as quickly as possible.

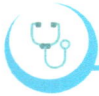

Electric shock

Effects can range from a tingle to cardiac arrest. There is no exact way to predict the injury from any given amperage. The table below shows generally how degree of injury relates to current passing through a body for a few seconds.

The effect of electric shock on the human body is determined by three main factors:

1. **How much current is flowing through the body (measured in amperes and determined by voltage and resistance).**

2. **The path of current through the body.**

3. **How long the body is in the circuit.**

Mild Shock
Trip setting for ground fault circuit interrupter

Muscle Contractions
Victim cannot let go

Severe Shock
Breathing difficult - possible respiratory arrest

Heart Stops pumping

Increasing probability of death

Enough current to light a 100 - watt bulb

INCREASING CURRENT

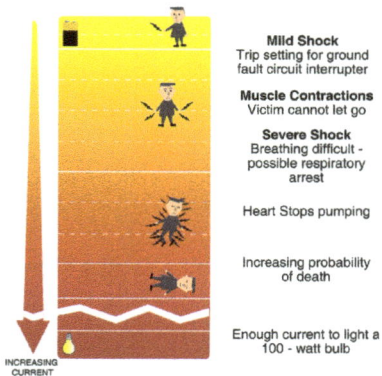

The above diagram shows the effect of electric shock on humans, but the effects are the same in cats.

Electrical injuries often affect the mouth as they are frequently due to *kittens* chewing electrical cables. The animal may have burns on the lips, tongue and across the roof of the mouth, so don't forget to open the mouth and have a look inside if you find a damaged electrical cable within your cat's reach. It is not unusual to find a burn line along the tongue of *kittens* prone to chewing cables.

If a high voltage supply is involved (non-domestic, for example, power lines), do not approach. Call the police.

In the home, turn off power first at the mains. If breathing and the heart has stopped, you may wish to give resuscitation. Call the vet immediately.

Electric shock, also referred to as electrocution, is most commonly seen in *kittens* and young cats after chewing electric cables, but can be seen in cats of all ages, sizes and breeds.

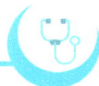

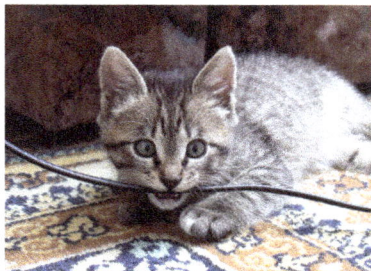

What is the effect of an electric shock?

A lot depends on the strength of the current, the voltage of the electricity and the duration of contact.

Very mild shocks may cause nothing more than mild discomfort similar to us experiencing a static build-up. However, even relative weak electrical currents can cause extensive burns as the current spreads through the tissues and causes them to overheat. Often the extent of the damage is not fully apparent until several days afterwards as the damaged tissue dies and forms ulcers. These can get infected very easily, and if in the mouth may be noticed as mouth pain or a foul smell.

Electricity can cause internal damage as the electricity travels through the body, in addition it often affects the heart which may cause your cat to collapse and could cause the heart to stop. Lightning strikes are usually immediately fatal.

How will I know if my cat has received an electric shock?

Cats may be found chewing something electrical or may jump as if they have just received a static shock. It is not uncommon to find pets unconscious close to a source of electricity, often still in contact with the source of electricity. Animals who have received a lightning strike are found dead, often with charring or other burn marks present.

Alternatively, mild cases may not be discovered until a day or two later when your cat starts showing signs of pain or secondary infection of burns.

Electricity can cause muscular spasms which can cause the jaws to clamp shut around cables so

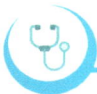

that they can't let go. The live current may still be present and will shock you too if you touch your cat, so the first step is to turn off the power if possible. The safest way to make the area safe is to turn off the power at the mains.

A cat showing any of the following signs needs urgent veterinary attention: evidence of burns, signs of pain or distress, increased drooling, irritation at the site of contact (e.g. pawing the mouth), coughing, breathing difficulties, collapse or unconsciousness.

Cats may show a delayed onset of signs as burns not obvious at the time become more apparent. Cats that have experienced a mild to moderate electric shock may show any or all of the following: pain at the site of shock (mouth pain, lameness etc.), coughing, difficulty eating, increased drooling or a foul odour to the breath. Pets showing these symptoms should be checked by a veterinary surgeon at the first possible opportunity.

Cats with breathing difficulties or heart rhythm abnormalities may deteriorate suddenly during the first few days. They require a high level of care in a veterinary hospital if they are to make a full recovery.

Prevention

Prevention is key: most electric shock injuries in the home are preventable. Cats should always be discouraged from chewing cables. Bitter tasting sprays from the pet shop can be useful to discourage chewing.

Always ensure that the area is safe if your pet has been electrocuted:

- Do not touch them until you have turned the electricity off at the mains. Electrical burns have an entry and exit and burn all the way through the inside. Therefore, the electrical burn is unlikely to be the most important injury and should not be a distraction, when they may be losing consciousness and could stop breathing as a result of the shock affecting their heart.

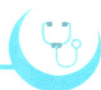

Poisoning

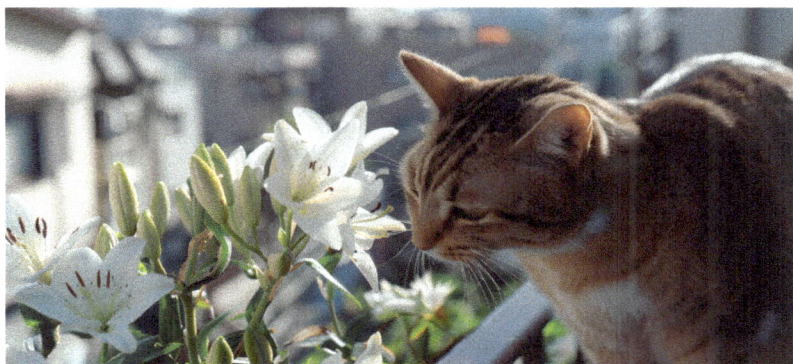

A poison is any substance (a solid, liquid, or a gas) which can cause damage if it enters the body in sufficient quantities.

A poison can be swallowed, breathed in, absorbed through the skin or injected.

Some poisons cause an all over reaction: and can result in seizures, blurred vision, acute anaphylaxis and can be fatal – be cautious and always get your cat quickly seen by a Vet

Many foods eaten regularly by humans, can be extremely dangerous to cats. Know the most common ones and keep them well out of reach and inaccessible to your pet.

Be aware that some substances have a delayed response in animals and they may not show signs of poisoning for hours or even days after they have eaten them.

If you suspect that your pet has eaten something not meant for them, always consult your Vet immediately for advice. Do not wait for symptoms.

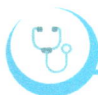

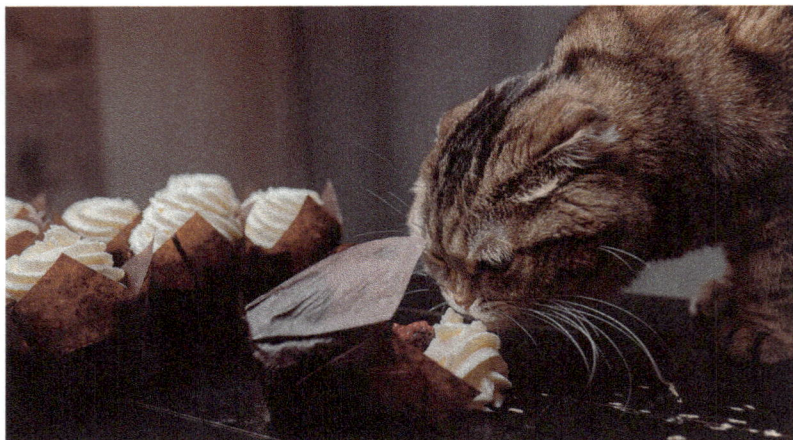

Prevention

The Royal Society for the Prevention of Cruelty to Animals RSPCA has some very useful advice on what to do if you suspect your cat is poisoned.

Keep dangerous substances out of reach

Keep all potentially harmful substances out of reach of your pets and ideally in a locked cupboard. This includes; sweets, dishwasher tablets, grapes and raisins, medicines – in particular Ibuprofen and any other sugar coated pills, alcohol, cosmetics, DIY, cleaning and gardening products.

Mindful about substances

Ensure that visitors understand how important it is not to leave potentially hazardous substances within reach – the contents of many handbags could be lethal to animals! Often visitors bring edible gifts such as chocolates and biscuits; cats can swiftly get through packaging.

Use original containers

Never decant medication or other products into different containers, always use the original containers, clearly labelled, with childproof / pet proof lids if possible.

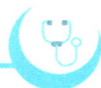

Batteries

Keep batteries out of reach of cats and small children and ensure that batteries in children's toys are firmly secured.

Check smoke alarms regularly

Fit carbon monoxide alarms and have appliances and alarms regularly checked. Pets and humans will both be adversely affected by Carbon Monoxide.

Harmful plants

Be aware of harmful plants – many decorative plants (particularly berry bearing Christmas plants) are toxic. Plants can be checked through the Royal Horticultural Society rhs.org.uk or by asking your local florist or horticultural nursery. Conkers and acorns can make your cat seriously ill.

Many human foods can be lethal to your pet

Chocolate, grapes, raisins, onions, artificial sweeteners and diet foods containing Xylitol are all potentially lethal. Ensure your pet is unable to access your rubbish / left overs, that could easily contain any of these foodstuffs.

Avoid your pet drinking from puddles that could be contaminated by Antifreeze. Antifreeze (Ethylene Glycol) is sweet and they love it – however unless they are treated by the Vet immediately, it can prove lethal.

Rock salt is poisonous to your pet, they usually make themselves ill by licking it from their paws when they get in from a walk – to prevent this, in winter time, always rinse and wipe their paws when they get home from their walk.

Be extremely careful that your cat does not ingest slug and snail pellets (containing Metaldehyde) and rat poison. If they eat something that has been poisoned, they will be affected by the poison too. Eating slug and snail pellets is one of the most frequent causes of poisoning death in pets.

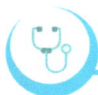

Common poisons – human food

There are many substances commonly available in the human world that can prove lethal to your pet. Always contact your Vet immediately if you suspect that your pet has ingested anything that could do them harm. Never watch and wait, many symptoms can take hours or days to manifest and by that time it could be too late.

Chocolate

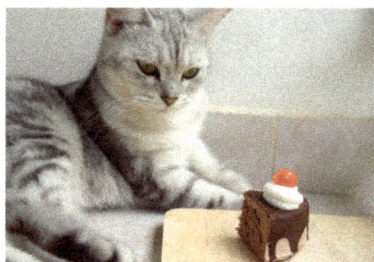

Chocolate contains a stimulant called Theobromine (similar to caffeine) that is poisonous to cats. The amount of Theobromine differs in the different types of chocolate (dark chocolate has the most in it and white chocolate has very little).

What does Theobromine do and what symptoms will I see?

Theobromine mainly affects the heart, central nervous system and kidneys. Symptoms will occur from 4-24 hours after your cat has eaten chocolate and will vary depending on the amount of chocolate (Theobromine) your cat has eaten.

If your cat has eaten chocolate, you may see the following symptoms, your cat is likely to have worse symptoms the more chocolate they have eaten and eating large amounts can prove fatal:

- **Vomiting (possibly including blood)**

- **Diarrhoea**

- **Hyperactivity and restlessness**

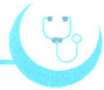

- **Rapid breathing**

- **Muscle twitching**

- **Increased heart rate**

- **Seizures / fitting**

If your cat has eaten any chocolate contact your Vet as quickly as possible with as much information as you can about how much they have eaten and the type of chocolate consumed. Preserve wrappers and remains of the chocolate and take them with you to the Surgery.

There is no antidote to Theobromine. In most cases your vet will initially make your cat vomit, wash out their stomach and then feed them activated charcoal to absorb any Theobromine left in the intestine.

(Please note that not all pets react to poisons in the same way and some appear to tolerate grapes, raisins and chocolate with no apparent ill- effects – there is no way to predict the effect these foods will have on your cat and so it is always best to avoid them)

Onions

Onions are toxic to cats and cats. Worryingly signs of poisoning occur a few days after consumption and so you may not be immediately aware of what is making your pet ill.
All forms of onion will make your pet ill including; dried / dehydrated, raw and cooked, so be particularly careful when disposing of left overs such as pizzas, Chinese and Indian food and even baby food often contains puréed onion.

The onion family causes gastrointestinal upset and may result in red blood cell damage, you should be particularly careful to keep these out of animal's reach.

Grapes and raisins

These fruits can be extremely dangerous to cats and the signs and symptoms may not become apparent for up to 5 days after consumption. Grapes and raising can cause kidney failure and are extremely dangerous to your pets. Contact your Vet if you suspect they have eaten them, even if your Pet seems fine.

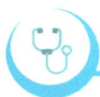

Macadamia nuts

Macadamia nuts cause cats to experience weakness, depression, tremors, vomiting and reduces their ability to maintain their body temperature and they may overheat. Symptoms typically last for approximately 12 to 48 hours – contact a Vet for further advice.

Alcohol

Alcohol is significantly more toxic to cats than to humans and may cause vomiting, diarrhoea, decreased coordination, depression of the central nervous system, shaking, difficulty breathing, abnormal blood acidity, coma and even death.

Caffeine

Cats are more sensitive to the effects of caffeine than people and large quantities can cause similar problems to chocolate toxicity.

Corn on the cob and sweetcorn

Cats are unable to easily digest corn on the cob and it often results in gastrointestinal blockage and causes constipation, vomiting and can make them very ill.

Xylitol

Xylitol is an artificial sweetener found in many foods such as sugar free gum, diabetic cakes and diet foods. This substance causes many animals to release insulin which can cause a potentially fatal lowering of their blood sugar (hypoglycaemia). Symptoms include lethargy, vomiting and loss of coordination, an inability to stand and seizures. Xylitol has also been linked to fatal acute liver disease and blood clotting disorders in cats. Even very small amounts can be extremely dangerous so contact your Vet immediately if worried.

Bones

Cooked bones are particularly dangerous for cats as the bones become brittle and can splinter causing choking or possibly puncturing further down the digestive tract. Small bones can get stuck in their bowel and often cause constipation.

Avocado

Avocados contain a substance called Persin contained in

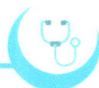

avocados which can cause vomiting and diarrhoea in cats.

Milk

Milk and milk products can cause diarrhoea in d as they struggle to break down lactose in milk.

Ibuprofen

Sugar coated Ibuprofen tablets are very appealing to cats – if you suspect they have eaten them you need to get immediate veterinary help. Symptoms include vomiting, diarrhoea, bleeding from the gut, stomach ulceration and kidney failure.

Tip : Always take the packaging and remains with you to the Vet as this will help them to estimate how much has been ingested and establish exactly what it was and if there is an antidote.

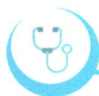

Common poisons - non-foods

There are many substances commonly available in the human world that can prove lethal to your pet.

Always contact your Vet immediately if you suspect that your pet has ingested anything that could do them harm.

Never watch and wait, many symptoms can take hours or days to manifest and by that time it could be too late.

Antifreeze

Prevent your cat from drinking from roadside puddles as these are often contaminated with antifreeze. Antifreeze (ethylene glycol) is sweet and very appealing to cats. There is an antidote (IV ethanol!), but it needs to be given immediately otherwise the effects are likely to be fatal.

Symptoms of Antifreeze poisoning include drunken behaviour, nausea and vomiting, diarrhoea, excessive urination, seizures, shaking and tremors, coma and death. It is an extremely common fatal poison.

Rock salt

Rock salt is a mixture of salt (sodium chloride) and grit, and is used to help de-ice roads in winter. Rock salt poisoning usually occurs in pets such as cats and cats when they lick it from their paws or fur when they return home.

Eating Rock Salt results in a high blood sodium concentration which can cause thirst, vomiting and lethargy, and in severe cases: convulsions and kidney damage. Seek Veterinary advice immediately.

Mouse and rat poison that is anticoagulant (eg Warfarin) based

If a cat eats rat poison or a rat or mouse that has been poisoned using an anticoagulant rodenticide such as Warfarin they

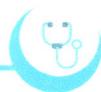

will be affected by the poison and it can make them extremely ill.

Warfarin Poisoning may cause life-threatening bleeding; effects may not appear for several days. Bleeding may be internal and is not always visible.

If caught early enough, your Vet may be able to treat them with vitamin K and they can make a full recovery. Always contact your Vet if there is a possibility they may have ingested rat poison, even if they are not as yet showing any symptoms.

Slug and Snail bait / poison

Metaldehyde is commonly found in slug/snail baits or pellets. Metaldehyde poisoning is extremely serious and is usually fatal without urgent treatment. Cats may initially appear unsteady on their feet and twitchy, but may rapidly deteriorate, suffering continuous seizures and difficulty breathing.

Ibuprofen

Sugar coated Ibuprofen tablets are very appealing to cats – if you suspect they have eaten them you need to get immediate veterinary help. Symptoms include vomiting, diarrhoea, bleeding from the gut, stomach ulceration and kidney failure.

Vitamin D

Vitamin D exists in many forms and is found in a variety of products and human skin creams.

Vitamin D Poisoning can cause vomiting, diarrhoea, bleeding from the gut, convulsions, abnormal heart rhythm and kidney failure. Effects may be delayed for several days and your pet may not recover.

Conkers and acorns and many plants

Conkers, acorns and many common plants have the potential to make your cat extremely ill. Always contact the Vet if at all worried.

Always take the packaging and remains with you to the Vet as this will help them to estimate how much has been ingested and establish exactly what it was and if there is an antidote.

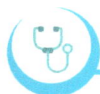

Breaks and Dislocations

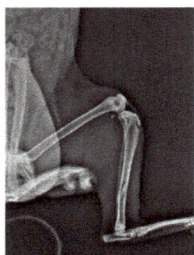

How do you know if they have broken a bone?

The honest answer is that unless the bone is sticking out, or the limb is at a very peculiar angle, the only way to know for sure that a bone is broken is to have an X-ray. A fracture is another word for a broken bone.

Other possible signs:

- **P**ain – it hurts

- **L**oss of power, it can be hard to move a broken limb

- **U**nnatural movement – the limb may be at an odd angle and have a wider range of movement than it should have

- **S**welling, bruising or a wound around the fracture site

- **D**eformity- often limbs may be shortened, or the broken area could have lumps and bumps or stepping (with an injured spine it is uneven as you gently feel down their back)

- **I**rregularity – lumps, bumps, depressions, or stretched skin

- **C**repitus – the grinding sound when the end of bones rub against each other

- **T**enderness – pain at the site of injury

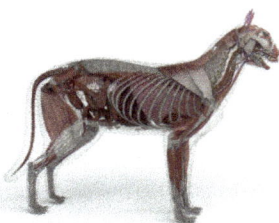

Important things to note with broken bones

Broken bones on their own, rarely cause fatalities. However, if there is severe bleeding associated with the injury

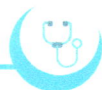

(either internal or external bleeding) this can cause the casualty to go into shock, which is life threatening.**

Do not attempt to reposition the injured limb.

Keep your pet warm and dry and be aware that pain and stress will adversely affect their condition.

If you are at all worried about them, phone your vet.

Types of Fractures

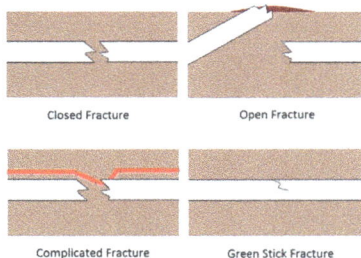

Closed Fracture   Open Fracture

Complicated Fracture   Green Stick Fracture

Open fractures - Phone for veterinary advice.

If the bone is sticking out, the bone is broken!

Be very aware of the onset of shock – keep them warm and dry, do not move or reposition the injured limb.

Complicated fractures - With complicated fractures, muscles, nerves, tendons and blood vessels could be trapped and damaged.

Keep them calm, warm and as still as possible and phone your nearest vet.

Do not attempt to splint or bandage the injured limb as you could make things worse.

Closed and greenstick fractures - The only sure way to tell if the bone is broken is to get it X-rayed.

Treating broken bones

Protect yourself and the animal from any further danger.

If you suspect that your pet has broken a limb. Do not try and reposition the limb and only apply a bandage if there is profuse bleeding that you need to control. Move the limb as little as possible. Make the animal as comfortable as possible and safely transported to the Vet for an x-ray.

Do not try and splint the limb, just comfortably transport your pet as quickly as possible.

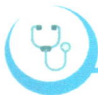

Dislocation

A dislocation occurs when the bone is pulled out of position at a joint and it can be accompanied by other tissue damage.

Always go to a Vet to replace a dislocated joint. Never try and put it back yourself as you are likely to cause further damage and trap nerves or blood vessels.

Signs and symptoms

They may have:

- difficulty moving the joint, pain and stiffness

- welling and bruising around the joint

- They are likely to be asymmetrical, with one joint looking deformed and out of place

- There could be shortening, bending or twisting of the joint

Treatment

- Keep everyone safe – muzzle your cat if there is a risk of being bitten

- Support the injury to avoid unnecessary and painful movement

- Never try and reposition the limb yourself

- Look out for signs of shock

- Phone the Vet and transport them carefully to your local Veterinary Clinic

- Do not allow them to eat or drink as they may need a general anaesthetic

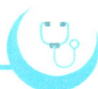

Head Injuries

Head injuries in cats can be extremely serious.

Phone a local Vet immediately, keep the animal warm and carefully transport them to the Veterinary Surgery. All pets that have experienced a head injury should be checked by a Vet.

A bang on the head can cause them to have a seizure

If they have a seizure, you should protect them from further danger, phone the Vet; dim lights and remain as quiet as possible whilst the seizure continues, put them in the recovery position once the seizure finishes (ref seizure section)

Head wounds can bleed profusely - don't panic!

The head and face are extremely vascular and consequently bleed profusely. Try not to panic, you will probably find that once you have applied firm pressure for 10 minutes that the wound is not nearly as bad as you feared.

Always call your Vet

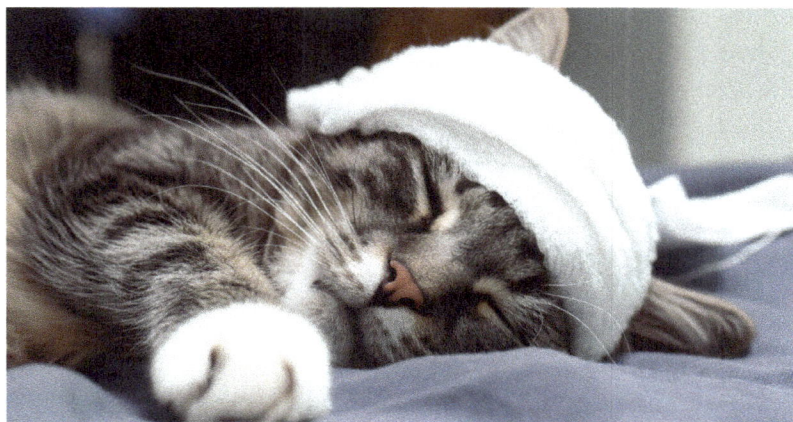

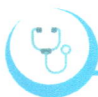

Spinal Injuries

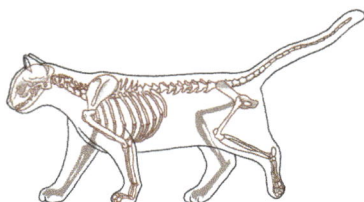

best not to twist their spine as you move them. A car parcel shelf or stiff board can be helpful as an improvised stretcher.

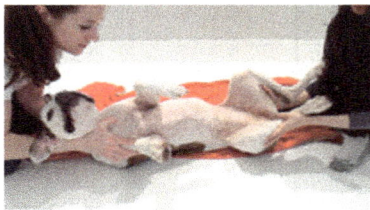

You should consider a spinal injury if:

- **They have fallen from more than twice their height, or been pushed with force**

- **Something heavy has fallen onto them,**

- **They have been involved in a road traffic accident – either within a moving vehicle, or being hit by anything at speed.**

- **They have a head injury.**

If they are conscious, keep them as still and calm as possible. Phone the Vet immediately, carefully transport to the closest Veterinary Surgery doing your

Ideally it is at least a two person job, with one person supporting the head and neck and the other coordinating the rest of the body to minimise twisting.

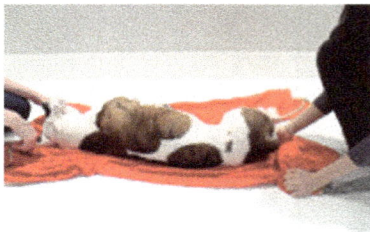

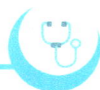

Seizures

Normal EEG

Parietal Lobe Frontal Lobe
Occipital Lobe
Cerebellum Temporal Lobe

Partial Seizure EEG

Generalized Seizure EEG

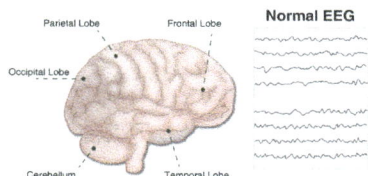

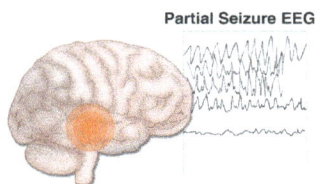

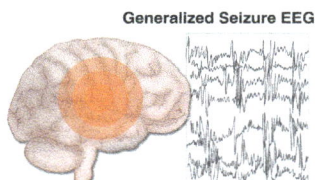

What is a seizure and why does it happen

A seizure (the medical term for a fit or convulsion) occurs when there is a sudden burst of electrical activity in the brain which causes a temporary disruption in the normal messaging processes. Seizures occur as a result of abnormal electrical activity within the brain that cause your cat's muscles to contract and relax rapidly.

Observation

Seizures can be partial or focal type; initially affecting certain parts of the brain and can then become generalized – observing how your pet behaves during a seizure can be helpful to the Vet and aid the diagnosis.

Many different types of seizures and different causes

The brain affects the whole of the body and so where the seizure occurs in the brain, will affect different parts of the body.

There are many different types of seizures and loads of different causes: any head injury or stress to the brain can cause fitting; as can brain tumours, poisoning, low blood sugar levels, calcium deficiency lack of oxygen, kidney or liver disease, raised body temperature eg heat stroke or infection, stroke, epilepsy...

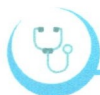

Epilepsy

A diagnosis of epilepsy is made when there has been at least one unprovoked seizure – that cannot be attributed to any other cause. It can be difficult to control epileptic seizures in cats.

What does a seizure look like?

Fits, seizures or convulsions can cause your pet to collapse and then experiencing rigid out of control movements. There may be absence seizures, where your pet is rigid and unresponsive, or full thrashing around tonic/clonic fits – or anything in between.

What to do

Cats can experience fits, convulsions or seizures for a variety of reasons. Most seizures are over very quickly within 2-3 minutes. Ideally let your pet finish their convulsion before attempting to transport them.

Always consult your Vet. If there are multiple seizures in quick succession or the seizure lasts longer than 5 minutes – you should contact the Vet

immediately as they may need veterinary intervention to stop the seizure.

Whilst your pet is having a seizure there is a reduced oxygen supply to the brain and this is one of the reasons why prolonged and continuous seizures can be life threatening.

(KEEP YOUR HANDS CLEAR OF THEIR MOUTH AND NEVER PUT ANYTHING IN OR NEAR THEIR MOUTH DURING A SEIZURE)

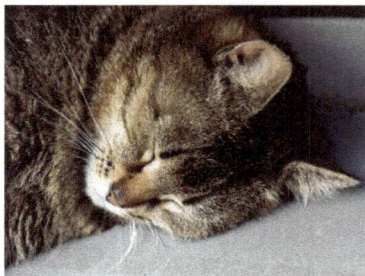

- During the seizure protect your pet from danger and anything against which they could hurt themselves – move furniture clear if necessary.

- Keep lighting low, noise to a minimum and avoid touching them too as external distractions can prolong a seizure.

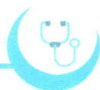

- Do not put anything in their mouth

- Make a note of the time the seizure started and exactly what happened – this may be useful for the Vet to diagnose the cause of the fit.

- Remove any objects they could hurt themselves against

- Once the seizure is over your pet could be disorientated for a while (possibly up to 2 hours), they are also likely to be thirsty so ensure they have easy access to drinking water.

- Never put your hand anywhere near a cat's mouth when it is having a seizure as it may involuntarily bite you

Call your Vet

There is a huge variety in the type of seizure, but often they begin with your cat trembling, their eyes glaze over and they don't respond to you and then may fall down and start to jerk violently. During a seizure it is common for them to urinate or defaecate and it is possible that they drool a lot and this could be blood stained if they have bitten their tongue.

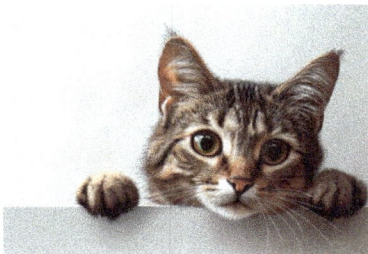

After the seizure, your cat may be disoriented or sleepy for up to a couple of hours.

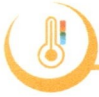

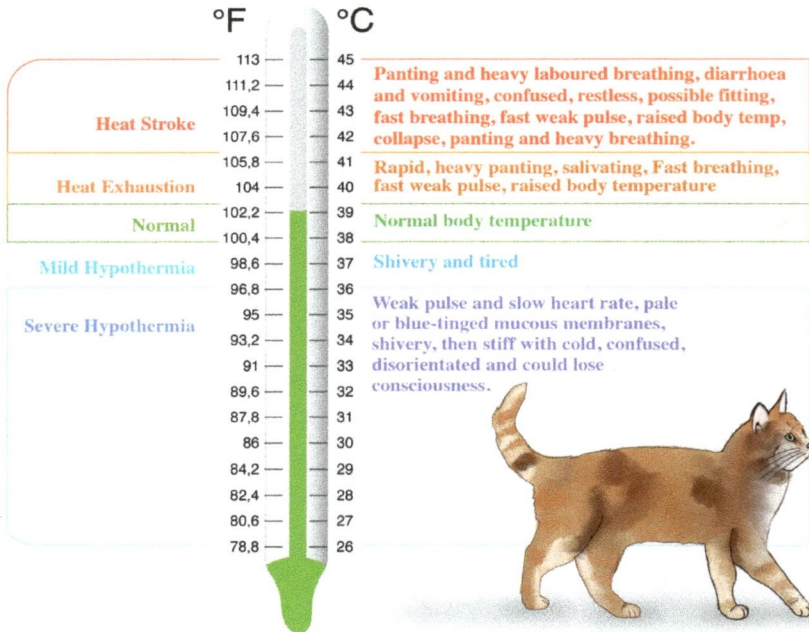

Extremes of body temperature

°F	°C	
113	45	
111,2	44	Panting and heavy laboured breathing, diarrhoea
109,4	43	and vomiting, confused, restless, possible fitting,
Heat Stroke 107,6	42	fast breathing, fast weak pulse, raised body temp, collapse, panting and heavy breathing.
105,8	41	Rapid, heavy panting, salivating, Fast breathing,
Heat Exhaustion 104	40	fast weak pulse, raised body temperature
Normal 102,2	39	Normal body temperature
100,4	38	
Mild Hypothermia 98,6	37	Shivery and tired
96,8	36	
95	35	Weak pulse and slow heart rate, pale
Severe Hypothermia 93,2	34	or blue-tinged mucous membranes, shivery, then stiff with cold, confused,
91	33	disorientated and could lose
89,6	32	consciousness.
87,8	31	
86	30	
84,2	29	
82,4	28	
80,6	27	
78,8	26	

Normal body temperature is between 38 deg C and 39.3 deg C (100.2-102.5 deg F)

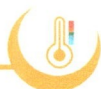

Heat Exhaustion

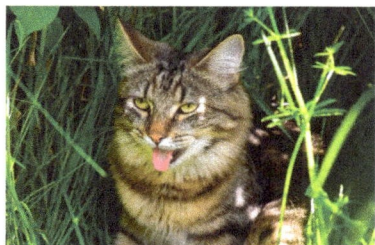

Cats are only able to lose heat by sweating from their nose and paws and panting.

They are therefore highly susceptible to overheating.

You should watch out for signs of heat exhaustion particularly if your cat is panting heavily and appears distressed on a hot day or after exercise. Short nosed cats (eg boxer, pug), older and overweight cats are particularly susceptible to getting over heated and out of breath when exercising.

Signs and symptoms:

- Rapid, heavy panting

- Salivating

- Fast breathing, fast weak pulse, raised body temperature

- Heat exhaustion occurs when their temperature rises over 39.3 and heat stroke over 41 degrees C.

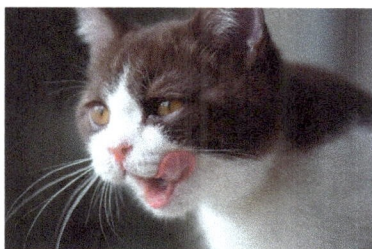

Heat stroke is a serious medical emergency and they will need urgent Veterinary help.

Prevention

- How to keep your cat cool and prevent heatstroke

- Make sure your cat has access to clean water at all times. Carry water and a bowl with you on walks.

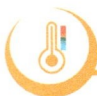

- Remember to have fresh water accessible on the beach too as drinking sea water will make them ill.

- On hot days, walk your cat during the cooler parts of the day, in the early morning and late evening

- Watch your pet for signs of over-heating, including heavy panting and loss of energy and if necessary, stop, find a shady spot and give your cat water.

Never leave your cat (or any pet) alone in a car, even with the windows open.

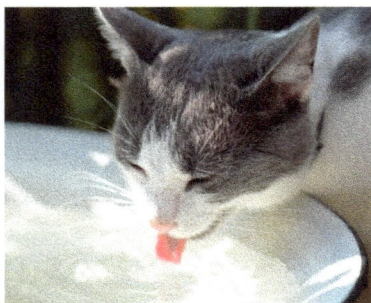

Treatment

- **Get urgent Veterinary advice.**

- Apply copious amounts of tepid water gently all over the cat and if available position near a fan to aid cooling.

- Ensure they have easy access to drinking water.

- Transport the cat to the Vet with car windows open and/or put on the air conditioning on.

- **NEVER immerse the cat in icy water as you may put them into shock.**

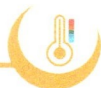

Heat Stroke

HEAT STROKE IS EXTREMELY SERIOUS – GET VETERINARY HELP FAST

Heat Stroke is a very serious condition when the body's temperature control mechanism fails and their temperature keeps rising to dangerously high levels – beyond 40C!

Signs and symptoms

- A very high temperature **>41 degrees**

- Panting and heavy laboured breathing

- Salivating, drawing back gums to expose more mucosal membrane

- Deep red sticky gums

- Have diarrhoea and vomiting

- Confused, restless and could start fitting.

- Fast breathing, fast weak pulse, raised body temperature

- Collapse

- Cats can suffer fatal heatstroke within minutes as unlike humans, cats can't sweat through their skin and so they rely on panting and releasing heat by sweating through their paw pads and nose to regulate their body temperature and keep cool.

- If you imagine wearing a thick winter coat on a hot summer's day and you'll understand why cats succumb to heatstroke so easily.

- **NEVER muzzle a cat experiencing Heat Stroke as they will need to be able to pant**.

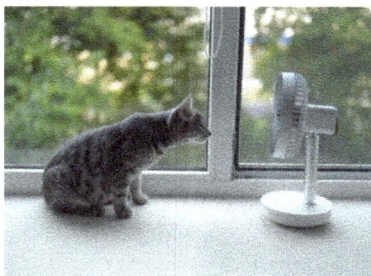

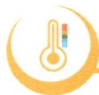

Hypothermia

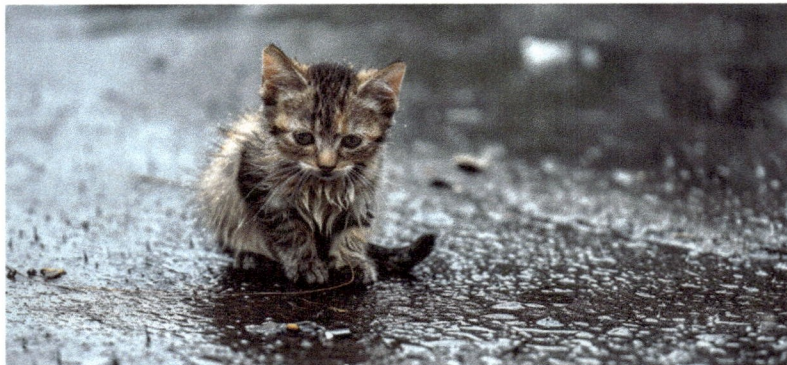

Hypothermia is defined as the point at which the core body temperature falls below 37C.

Hypothermia will occur if your cat gets too cold and is most common if they have been in freezing water, even for a few minutes.

Sick, very old and very young cats are less able to regulate their own body temperature and therefore more likely to get hypothermia. These cats may need a coat or sweater when taken out for walks in the winter. Extreme hypothermia is very serious and can be fatal.

Signs and symptoms

- Weak pulse and slow heart rate

- Dilated pupils

- Mucous membranes become pale or blue tinged.

- They may be shivery and then stiff with cold.

- As hypothermia develops further, they become confused, disorientated and then may lose consciousness – severe hypothermia kills.

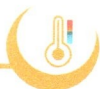

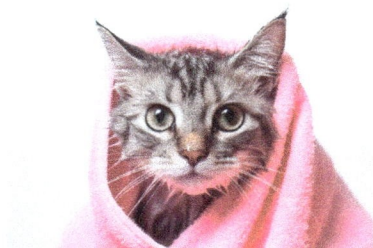

if they are very cold, keep them as still as possible as the extreme cold can affect their heart and any swift movement can cause a Cardiac Arrest.

Treatment

- Remove them from the cold. Wrap in warm dry clothing or a towel, blanket.

- Wrap up warm in coats and blankets, and increase the room temperature if possible as well

- Use your body warmth and wrapped warm water bottles to gently warm them through.

- A foil blanket can be helpful

- Get veterinary advice quickly.

- If they lose consciousness and are breathing – put in the recovery position,

- If they stop breathing – do CPR

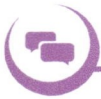

When is it an emergency?

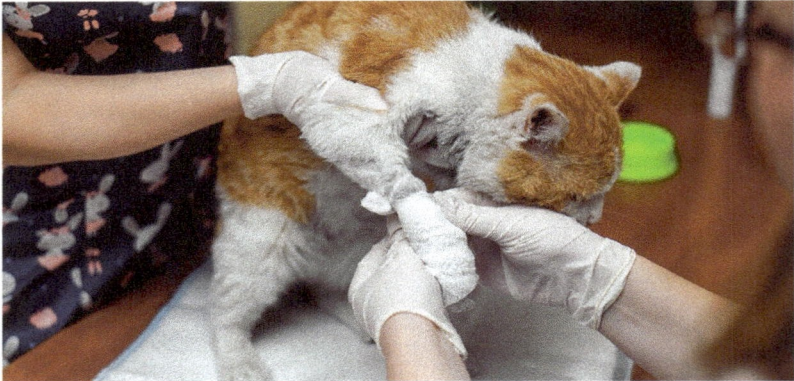

When your pet has an accident or is ill it can be incredibly difficult to assess how serious it is and whether it is necessary to involve the Vet. Our advice would always be to seek veterinary advice and they will be able to talk things through and help you to make the right choice.

The following information aims to help you with this extremely important decision:

The decision will vary from case to case, but we would strongly advise that the following constitutes a veterinary emergency:

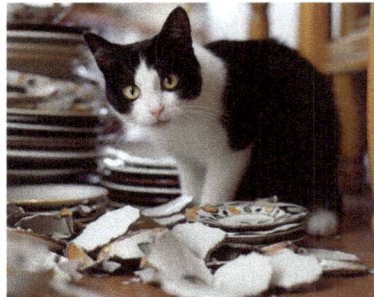

- Appears not to be breathing, is struggling for breath or breathing in a strange way.

- If they have a severe injury that is bleeding profusely and you are unable to stop with direct pressure on the wound

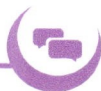

- If they are unconscious or unaware of what is going on around them.

- If they are having a severe allergic reaction.

- If they are burnt and their skin is visibly damaged or blistered.

- If they have fallen from a height, been hit by something traveling at speed (like a car) or been hit with force.

- If you suspect they have ingested antifreeze, rat poison or any other poisonous substance.

- They appear to have severe abdominal pain, a bloated stomach and attempt to vomit – bringing up white foam – this could be a sign of bloat (Gastric Dilation Volvulus GDV) which is extremely dangerous and potentially fatal.

- If they have an extremely high or low temperature it is a Veterinary emergency.

- If your pet has an eye injury they should be seen immediately by a Vet.

- All bite wounds should be checked, cleaned and dressed by a Vet.

- Deep wounds should be properly cleaned and dressed by a Vet.

- If your cat has recovered from a near drowning experience they should be checked by a Vet to prevent secondary drowning.

- If they have had a seizure and seem to have made a full recovery, it is always sensible to get them checked out.

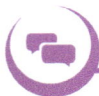

Caring for a neonate

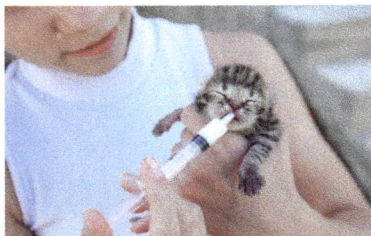

Caring for newborn kittens and puppies (neonates)

It is a sad fact that even with the best care, some abandoned and newborn kittens and puppies may not survive. However, this information should help you give a newborn kitten or puppy a really good chance.

The key threats to the neonates are hypothermia (low body temperature). dehydration and hypoglycaemia (low blood sugar). These problems are interrelated and may occur at the same time in one or more of the neonates.

If you find abandoned kittens or puppies, contact your Vet and no-kill shelters to see if they have a nursing mother cat or dog to adopt them, or experienced volunteers available to offer advice or even help bottle feed them.

Heat and bedding for newborn kittens and puppies

Neonates are unable to maintain their own body temperature and this can be life-threatening. From the moment you find them, keep the neonates warm and watch out for signs of chilling (i.e., listlessness and cool to the touch). If you have nothing else on hand, use your own body heat to warm up a cold kitten or puppy, and rub them gently to aid circulation. If they are cold, rewarm gradually over 30 to 60 minutes. Warming them too rapidly could prove fatal.

Neonates cannot control their body temperature until they are at least 3 weeks old.

During the first four days of a puppy or kitten's life, they should be maintained in an environmental temperature of 85° to 90F (29.4° to 32.2°C). The temperature may gradually be decreased to 80°F (26.7°C) by the

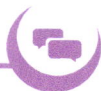

seventh to tenth day and to 72°F (22.2°C) by the end of the fourth week. If the litter is large, the room or environmental temperature need not be as high. As neonates huddle together, their body heat provides additional warmth.

At home, build a soft nest with a heating pad that is completely covered with a blanket or towel. Make sure that neonates can move away from the heat if they want. Change the bedding daily or when they have accidents. A neonate can chill if she gets wet, so never submerge them in water.

If they need to be cleaned, only wash the essential areas with a cloth and ensure you fully dry with a hair dryer (on low) and towel.

Kittens and puppies are most vulnerable during their first 24 hours.

What do you need to do for newborn kittens or puppies?

Identify each kitten or puppy: You'll need to monitor each kitten individually. A simple way to ensure you recognise them is to create collars using different colours of wool for each one. Remember to change these for bigger collars as they grow.

Weigh each neonate: The growth rate between birth and two days old is an important health indicator in neonatal care, so it's important to record their birth weight, followed by daily recordings of their weight to track their progress. Use digital scales to take accurate measurements within 1g and make sure they're clean and disinfected. Healthy neonates should double their birth weight in the first two weeks, then continue to gain weight steadily.

Examine from head to tail:

Keep a close eye on the development of each neonate. If they aren't gaining weight, if you are concerned about any potential abnormalities, or if you believe something is wrong with them, seek immediate advice from your vet.

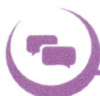

Feeding and looking out for signs of dehydration

Although neonates are born without sight and can't stand, within the first hours they'll begin to crawl to the mother's teats. There's usually some competition among siblings and they'll each choose a nipple they prefer to suckle from within the first three days. Make sure all the neonates are suckling regularly to get the nutrients they need to grow.

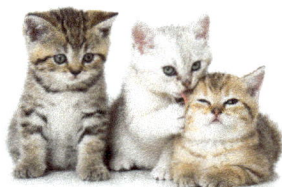

If the mother is struggling to feed her offspring, they don't seem to be receiving enough milk, or they have been abandoned, you may be required to support them with appropriate neonate milk substitutes. Always use a proper milk substitute as other alternatives can cause diarrhoea and make them ill.

Growth: Even by one day old the neonate should have begun to grow. Healthy neonates must gain weight on a daily basis. If they don't gain weight, or if they lose weight in the first few days, they should be checked by a vet to make sure there's no underlying illness.

Ideally the mother cat should stay with her offspring and begin licking them. This not only cleans them and provides comfort; it encourages them to suckle and stimulates them to defecate and urinate.

Dehydration

Two common signs of dehydration are the loss of elasticity in the skin and dry and sticky gums in the mouth. If they are dehydrated, their skin will fail to immediately spring back to its normal position after being pulled or and the gums will feel 'tacky' or clammy when touched. Testing their gums is the best measure of dehydration as very young puppies and kittens do not usually have the same skin elasticity as adults.

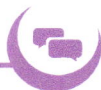

An environmental relative humidity of 55 to 65 percent is adequate to prevent drying of the skin in a normal neonate. However, a relative humidity of 85 to 90 percent is better if they are small and weak. Place a warm, wet washcloth in their box to help maintain a high humidity. Be sure to remove the wet cloth once it cools since a wet cloth can cause up to 25 percent more heat loss than air. A humidifier is also an excellent tool to maintain proper humidity for the neonates.

Caution: The environmental or external temperature should not exceed 90°F (32.2°C) when high humidity is provided. A temperature of 95°F (35.0°C) coupled with relative humidity of 95 percent can lead to breathing difficulties.

Hypoglycaemia:

Neonatal puppies and kittens are also at risk of low blood sugar level that can lead to severe depression, lethargy, 'sleepiness' or inactivity, muscle twitching, seizures and convulsions.

If a puppy or kitten shows signs of hypoglycemia, you should give them a solution containing glucose (such as corn syrup) and contact your Vet.

Signs there could be a problem:

- No weight gain during the first two days.

- Constant crying.

- Always consult your vet if you believe that the mother isn't feeding sufficiently.

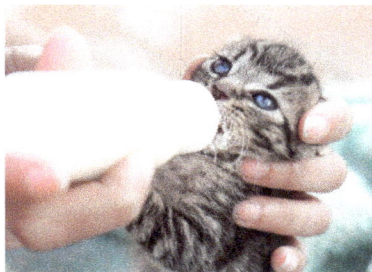

How to feed a newborn kitten or puppy:

If you need to begin bottle-feeding a neonate there are some important things to remember.

Use specific milk formula designed for puppies or kittens - never give cow's milk, goats milk,

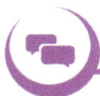

human baby formula or dairy alternatives. They don't provide the nutrients they need and may upset their stomach.

For neonatess suckling properly, a kitten bottle with the right sized teat is the safest way to feed. A syringe may be better for some kittens under 10 days old, or an eye dropper.

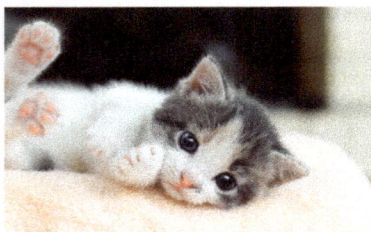

Keep the neonate is in an upright position, or on their front while feeding. They must not be on their back.

Feed very slowly, one drop at a time, to avoid the risk of the kitten breathing in the fluid.

Take great care with hygiene.

Keep your hands and the feeding equipment scrupulously clean, infection is a huge risk to them, sterilise everything as much as possible. Make a fresh portion for each feed, discarding any unused milk afterwards.

Feeding Frequency

10 days or younger every two hours around the clock

11 days to 2½ weeks every three to four hours

2½ to 4 weeks every five to six hours

4 weeks and older two to three times a day.

From 3 to 4 weeks you can start mixing formula with wet food and encourage them to lap it up, or put the mixture in a bottle. Then mix with dry food and begin providing it with water.

After Feeding
How to Burp a neonate

As long as they are drinking formula, you will have to burp them. Put them on your shoulder or on their stomachs and pat them gently until you feel them burp. Formula is sticky, so be sure to clean them after feeding with a warm, damp washcloth, and dry them with a towel.

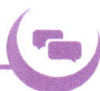

Elimination

Kittens and puppies under 4 weeks must be stimulated in order to go to poo and wee after each feeding. Use a warm, moist cotton ball, tissue, or washcloth to gently rub the kittens' anal area to stimulate urination and defecation.

When do they start to eat from a bowl?

From three to 4 weeks, they can start to eat food from a dish along with the milk replacer. A gruel can be made by thoroughly mixing canned or dry food (suitable for puppies or kittens) with the milk replacer to reach the consistency of a thick milk shake. The mixture should not be too thick or they will not eat very much. As they begin to eat more, you can reduce the amount of milk replacer.

Start house training at 4 weeks.

Some kittens may start looking for a place to go as young as 2½ weeks old. Use a small, shallow litter pan with non-clumping litter. Do not add paper or fabric as this can teach bad habits. Show kittens the litter box and add in a used cotton ball. They should learn what to do.

For puppies, take them out every hour during the day and 30 minutes after they have eaten to establish good habits. As they grow, they should be able to hold on longer and they don't like being dirty. Use newspaper or puppy pads in their crate overnight so they have somewhere to go that you can clean up easily.

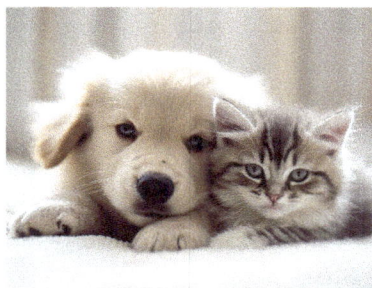

Health issues to look out for in newborn kittens and puppies

Incompatible blood groups

Neonatal isoerythrolysis can affect newborn kittens after suckling colostrum. It happens

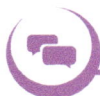

if they have a different blood group from their mother, as their red blood cells are destroyed by antibodies in the colostrum. Symptoms can range from haemorrhaging and death to anaemia, weight loss and weakness. Professional breeders select their stud cat and queen after completing a number of tests to be sure they have compatible blood groups.

Toxic milk syndrome

This bacterial infection is caused by kittens suckling from an infected mammary gland (a condition known as mastitis). Check the mother's teats for signs of inflammation and look out for weakening or lack of growth in the kitten. The milk may also be yellow-green or red-brown and the kitten may cry or have digestive difficulties.

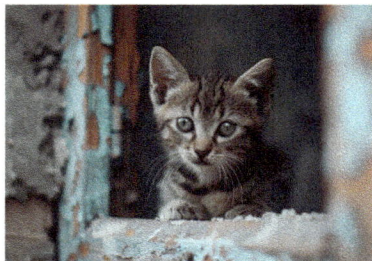

Upper Respiratory Infection (URI)

If they are coughing up phlegm, have a runny nose or trouble breathing or eating, consult your Vet immediately. A mild URI can be cleared up by wiping away discharge with a warm, wet cloth and keeping kittens in a warm, damp environment.

Fleas

Fleas on a very small kitten can cause anaemia. Pick fleas off with a flea comb. For a bad infestation, you can bathe the neonate in warm water and kitten or puppy shampoo. Avoid the eye area use a washcloth around the face and rinse them thoroughly.

Be sure to dry them after a bath so they do not chill. Do not use flea shampoo or topical flea treatments on kittens 6 weeks or younger.

Parasites

Kittens and puppies should begin a deworming treatment schedule as young as 10 days old; see a veterinarian for this. They tend to contract worms from their mother.

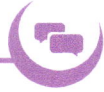

Diarrhoea

Diarrhoea is a serious condition. It may be caused by over feeding, giving too concentrated a solution of milk replacer, or be due to an infection (usually caused by poor hygiene). If they are experiencing diarrhoea, they should be taken to see a vet. Treatment must be swift as dehydration can then develop very rapidly.

When to contact your vet

Neonates are most vulnerable in the first few hours and days, so it's highly recommended to get them checked. If you feel something's not right with a newborn, always contact your Vet.

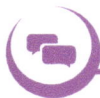

Behavioural changes

Key behaviour changes to look out for that could show you something is wrong:

- Changes in appetite and thirst

- Changes in bowel movements

- Changes in frequency and amount of urination

- Change in the way they smell

- Retreating and no longer wishing to socialise

- Lethargy

- Other signs of possible illness or injury:

- A distended and painful belly

- Diarrhoea and vomiting

- Limping

- Choking, retching or coughing

- Yelping or whining

- Discharge from eyes, ears, nose or rectum

- Difficulty breathing, wheezing or panting

- Bleeding

- Excessive scratching

- Disorientation, confusion or aggression

- Pacing

- Strange lumps

- Lack of responsiveness

- Any other change in behaviour that concerns you

Notes

Notes

www.ingramcontent.com/pod-product-compliance
Lightning Source LLC
Chambersburg PA
CBHW051259020426
42333CB00026B/3282